The Smallholder's Guide to Animal Ailments

Edited by
Russell Lyon BVM&S, MRC'

D1504845

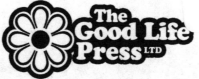

Published 2009 by The Good Life Press Ltd.

ISBN 9781904871514

A catalogue record for this book is available from the
British Library.

Published by
The Good Life Press Ltd.
PO Box 536
Preston
PR2 9ZY

www.goodlifepress.co.uk
www.homefarmer.co.uk

Design and layout by The Good Life Press Ltd.
Printed in the United Kingdom by Cromwell Press Group.

Contents

INTRODUCTION

Veterinary surgeons spend a minimum of five years and often much longer in training for their chosen profession. The average stockman/woman cannot be expected to match that level of knowledge when it comes to knowing about livestock ailments and disease conditions, especially when the vet concerned is mostly dealing with farm animals. Small animal vets will be able to cope with an emergency situation if really required as they have the necessary training, but most would really much prefer not to be "outside their comfort zone."

Part of the consideration about setting up even a limited livestock enterprise is to check whether there is locally a veterinary practice which deals regularly with farm animals and poultry and, if not, think again. Farm practices are now getting quite thin on the ground in some parts of the UK and the welfare of your livestock (eg. cow calving or sow farrowing etc.) might be severely at risk if the vet has to travel a long distance to reach your premises. In addition, the further a vet has to travel from his or her base, the more expensive it is for you the client.

The most important skill a stockperson must learn is the art of observation: time spent leaning over a gate just watching your stock while you get to know them and them you is not misspent. Knowing what is normal behaviour in an animal is vital. If you know what is normal behaviour then you will instantly know what is not. If you are not sure and lack experience by all means ask advice from an experienced person. However, if in doubt get in touch with your vet. Vets are usually quite happy to give advice over the telephone and will be able to decide from the information you can give from your observations, whether a visit is required.

It makes a lot of sense to reduce the time the vet has to spend on your premises by having good facilities on hand with which to catch and restrain the patient, or indeed the whole herd or flock if necessary. This is especially true for cattle, sheep and pigs. Cattle stocks or crushes can be expensive to buy new but can be obtained more reasonably second hand. Possession of stocks, races and pens, even those made temporarily with gates, are invaluable and will save the vet a great deal of time and you money. It's no good the vet turning up to be greeted by a casual "it's in the field, won't take us five minutes to catch it." It never does and it may cost you more for the visit.

Keeping livestock is a privilege and with it comes responsibilities and a duty of care. The Animal Welfare Act 2006 and the Welfare of Farm Animals 2007 make it an offence to cause unnecessary suffering to any animal and are designed to protect the welfare of all farm animals.

Welfare codes are available from Defra in booklet form for every species of farm animal. Copies of these codes are available from Defra and from the Stationary Office Publications Centre and everybody should have a copy relevant to the animals on their farm. These codes lay down minimum requirements for all farmed animals and cover specific requirements such as inspections, record keeping, freedom of movement, buildings and equipment and the feeding and watering of animals. It is important to remember that these codes are minimum requirements and most livestock owners or keepers should attempt an even higher standard of care than those demanded by legislation. Animal Health carries out welfare inspections (spot checks sometimes) on farms to check that legislation and the welfare codes are being followed. Defra has a contract with ADAS (an agricultural consultancy) to run an advisory programme to encourage good welfare and this advice is free! It's not often the Government gives something for nothing, so it makes sense to use the service. Subjects covered fairly recently include handling and condition scoring in cattle, mastitis in dairy cattle, improving calf, lamb and piglet survival, sheep kept on arable farms, poultry heat stress and litter management and pig housing systems. Just about something for everyone and the list is being added to all the time.

Keeping and rearing animals should not be about legislation, which is of course vital for the safety of farm animals, but should be pleasurable (apart from the obvious bad day now and again!) and very much a way of life. If it becomes a chore and only a means of making money (unlikely these days!), then it should be time to reassess the future of your livestock enterprise.

This is not a veterinary textbook but is written by practical people who are recognized to have a particular knowledge of the species about which they write. Some of the opinions expressed are individual and based on years of experience and will not necessarily coincide with accepted veterinary opinion. Given the knowledge obtained from this book and from your own experience there will be times when you will recognize a disease or condition in an animal and will wish to get it treated. Your vet has to be the first port of call for this, but do not expect the veterinary practice to be able to

supply the necessary drugs or treatment on request. The sale of medicines is strictly controlled into various categories, which the vet or pharmacist has to observe by law. Failure on their part to obey the legislation would have serious professional consequences for them.

Broadly speaking authorised veterinary medicine sales come into 4 different categories which were updated in 2008. These lay down guidelines for the dispensing, use and safe storage of all medicines.

AVM-GSL (authorised veterinary medicine – general sales list): Any outlet that cares to stock them may sell all medicines in this list. Vitamins and minerals are generally included.

NFA-VPS (non–food animal medicine – vet, pharmacist, suitably qualified person): In this category are medicines for non-food-producing animals such as companion animals. A vet, pharmacist or other suitably qualified person (such as a registered merchant) and no others can supply a medicine for a companion animal. This category may include some equine treatments if the animals themselves have been certified as not intended for human consumption. This was the former PML list or Merchant list category and mostly includes worming and anti-parasitic preparations.

POM–VPS (prescription only medicines - vet, pharmacist, suitably qualified person): Medicines in this category for food producing animals (including horses) can only be dispensed by the above people and only on receipt of a veterinary prescription, either orally or in writing. This list includes many medicines from the outdated Merchant list products (PML).

POM –V (prescription only medicines – vet only): Medicines in this category, which includes antibiotics, can only be supplied by a vet or by a pharmacist or another vet on receipt of a veterinary prescription. The vet can only dispense the medicines if the animals are under his or her care and following a clinical assessment. Livestock keepers must be aware of these very real constraints on vets who prescribe drugs in this category and should not be surprised or annoyed when their vet cannot supply many medications on demand. Most vets will insist on examining the animal(s) concerned before supplying medication if the animal has not been seen for at least 3 months or a new disease condition is suspected. Failure to do this by the vet concerned could have serious professional consequences for him or her, including being struck off by the Royal College of Veterinary Surgeons.

Any treatment given to your animal, whether by yourself or by the vet, has to be recorded and a record retained for inspection if required during a welfare inspection. You must be able to identify the treated animal and have recorded as a minimum requirement the withdrawal date of the drug before the meat, milk or eggs may enter the food chain.

Any animal you keep and rear for food or pleasure can become ill. Preventing disease by good husbandry and effective vaccination programmes makes good economic sense. This does not mean you have to use every vaccine known to man and livestock. Some are vital such as erysipelas vaccination for pigs, clostridia vaccination for sheep and goats and bluetongue vaccine for sheep, goats, cattle and deer. Using other available vaccines will depend on local conditions in your area and particular to your livestock unit. Your local vet is the best person to know this type of information and will willingly give advice, especially if you are intending to buy the vaccine, at least initially, from the veterinary practice.

One final thing to remember, as one of my old Fen farming clients was fond of saying,

was "when you have livestock you will have dead stock." It will happen, but it's how you deal with it that matters and if this book helps in any way to alleviate disease, suffering and premature death, it will have done its job.

Russell Lyon BVM&S, MRCVS
Suffolk 2009

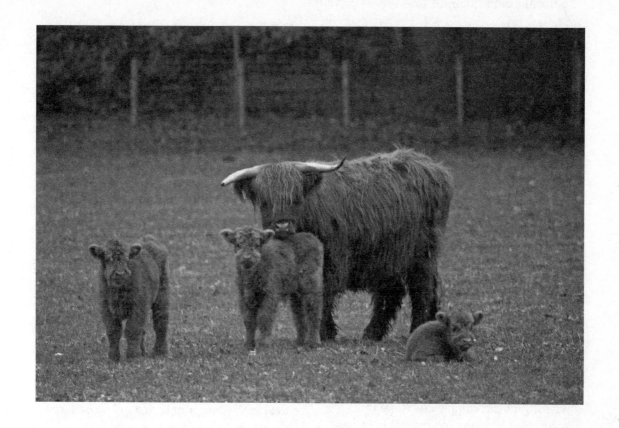

Chapter One

CATTLE HEALTH

By Peter King

Good stock management and the correct feeding regime will minimise health and disease risks in your animals, however you must be aware of potential problems so that you can react swiftly to any developing situations. The timing of your response to a situation is usually the critical factor when dealing with health and disease.

Cattle can be affected by a number of diseases, but you will have to be very unlucky indeed to be confronted by most of them. However, you should get yourself a good general reference book to diseases of cattle so that you

can broaden your overall knowledge, as well as have some information to hand at times of concern.

You should also confer with your vet and ask him to help you prepare a written herd health plan. Having such a plan will help you to qualify for various 'Farm Assured' schemes, should you wish to join one. On a small scale this is a simple exercise, so do not be daunted.

The type of health plan you draw up will be dictated by how much land is available, stocking density and whether you are taking the organic 'route' as certain restrictions on the type, application and withdrawal period of medicines apply to organic systems. If you are going organic you can apply for dispensations to use normally restricted medicines to deal with endemic problems which may affect your holding. Contact your certification body for more details. Your vet will also be able to teach you how to give injections properly, as well as giving guidance on administering other treatments.

Local Health Problems

It is always a good idea to gain as much local knowledge from your neighbours as you can. Your vet will also have specialised local knowledge of potential problems. There may even be hazards specific to your holding: old cattle sheds may harbour ringworm, a fungal skin disease, and no amount of cleansing may solve the problem completely. Rotavirus, which causes scouring (diarrhoea) in calves, may also be difficult to remove completely. On occasion, rotavirus may only be controlled through routine use of a vaccine if it is 'endemic' on the farm. This type of routine treatment would not lead to the removal of organic status if it is a recognised problem.

Accidents and Prevention

If potential hazards on your holding have been minimised, then accidents should be a very rare occurrence.

• Always keep gates to the road closed just in case the animals escape from the field into your yard.

• Always clear away any netting, barbed wire or sections of baling twine (which cattle and in particular calves seem to love to chew, and worse, swallow).

• It may be worthwhile removing broken thorny hawthorn branches and twigs during routine field inspections.

• Block off potential escape routes where an animal can damage itself.

• Rabbit burrows and any other holes in the path of the animals should be filled in. A broken leg can mean the end for an animal. (I have seen cows with false legs, but you need to be quite wealthy!)

First Aid

Even on the tidiest holding the occasional accident is unavoidable – the animals cannot be watched 24 hours a day. While some injuries may result in the animal having to be put down, most minor injuries can be dealt with using simple first aid and you should be able to deal with some simple first aid procedures without calling on the vet or neighbours, at least in the first instance. A limping cow may only have a hawthorn twig stuck between her hooves. A calf with a piece of baling twine dangling from its mouth may not have swallowed it too far, so it should be easy enough to remove. Cuts and rips to the skin can be treated with iodine or an antiseptic spray, which should be part of your first aid kit, but note that it does sting so you won't get any thanks. Any of these simple procedures are easier to deal with if you can coax the patient into a confined handling area as described. If this is not possible, then stealth is your best ally; reassuring words, stroking the animal and a little food, followed by speedy action Having a good relationship with your cattle is always a real help in any first aid situation.

Below is a basic list and your vet may advise the inclusion of additional items. Some items will need to be renewed as they pass their sell-by date. Just be glad you didn't need to use them!

- Digital thermometer
- Scour (diarrhoea) formula *(particularly if calf rearing)*
- Colostrum substitute *(optional)*
- Liquid iodine for wounds, navel dressing, disinfectant
- Magnesium and calcium solutions *(watch the sell-by dates; you must keep this in stock – by the time you have gone to get some when you need it, it could be too late when you get back)*
- 16 gauge x 1 inch hypodermic needles
- A quantity of 20ml syringes and a few 50ml
- Bandage and wound dressings
- Calving ropes and obstetric gel
- Washing soda crystals and/or peanut oil *(otherwise known as groundnut oil, which, if you cannot get it from your agricultural merchant, can be bought in litre bottles from retail food outlets)*
- Glucose powder
- Antiseptic spray
- Stomach tube kit
- Disinfectant
- Observation

Observation is the key word in managing the health of your stock. On a busy holding, particularly in winter when the days are short, you may be working flat out just to get all your jobs done, but you must include time to stand at the gate or at the pen, preferably twice or more times a day to avoid missing any important signals or potential problems. If you do this regularly you will be surprised how quickly you become attuned to the condition of your stock. Another benefit of this type of daily contact is that the animals respond to their keeper in a wholly positive way, strengthening the bond between man and beast.

In the field one of the most obvious signs that an animal is not feeling well is that it will stay away from you and the rest of the herd when you call them to you. It should be noted, however, that young calves may stay away from the gathering if they have only just woken up. If this happens it may still be wise to go and check on the calf anyway.

Temperature

The most significant indicator of an animal's health is its temperature, except for obvious problems such as eye infections. If you are concerned about an animal's overall demeanour it is a good idea to take its temperature. Your basic first aid kit includes a digital thermometer. They are not too expensive and are very easy to read. This is taken rectally. The normal body temperature for cattle is 38.5°C (101.5°F). Temperature can increase if a female is on heat, but as a general rule if there is any variance from normal temperature ie. if the temperature is lower or higher than normal for much longer than an hour or two and the animal is displaying other symptoms that are concerning you, then contact your vet, giving details of all the symptoms and the temperature of the animal in question. Continue to monitor the temperature regularly to see how things are going.

Isolation

Depending on the seriousness and potential infectivity of the ailment, you should always have a space to put your sick animal(s). This provides a warm, dry place for the patient, makes it easier to administer treatment and minimises the spread of infection. Although the animal may be stressed by being separated from the rest of the herd, with plenty of attention from you they could recover more quickly than if they were at the mercy of the elements.

If you suspect a contagious disease, separate the affected animal sooner rather than later. You can always let them out again if your suspicions prove unfounded.

Homeopathy

Many people now use homeopathy alongside conventional treatments, particularly organic producers. You may be fortunate enough to have a local vet who practices both conventional and alternative disciplines. Whatever your views on this it is vital to remember that an animal should not be made to suffer for the sake of ideological principles – the animal's welfare should always come first. I have , however, heard of a number of cases where it has been used to good effect in dairy herds, particularly for the treatment of mastitis.

AILMENTS AND DISEASES

Below are most of the more common disorders which can affect cattle, followed by a list of some less common diseases. It is recommended that you obtain a good cattle health reference to broaden your knowledge and help with diagnosis.

Hoof Care and Lameness

If an animal is limping it should demand your immediate attention. The likelihood is that it may just have a foreign object trapped or embedded in its foot. The damage caused by such objects can lead to a general complaint known as foul-in-the-foot or foot rot, which is caused when a wound becomes infected. If your animals are used to regular hoof inspections, a quick but careful inspection in the field may reveal and solve the problem, but when inspecting hooves, do not go straight to the foot as this will probably make the animal move away quickly. It is much better to greet them,

scratch the tailhead for a while and gradually work your way down, being aware that a kick might be forthcoming! If all your attempts at casual inspection fail, monitor the situation for 24 hours and, if there is no improvement, a thorough inspection should then be carried out, initially by you and, if necessary, your vet, by restraining the animal in a crush. If you do not have a cattle crush use your gates to make a narrow pen, preferably beneath a beam or branch so that you can use a rope to lift and restrain the leg to enable you to work safely. It can be difficult to see if an object has embedded itself and you may need professional help to diagnose and solve the problem fully.

It may be the long sward rather than a foreign object which has caused soreness between the claws, however it may be wise to give a precautionary injection of penicillin. Your vet will advise you on this. If the lameness is due to an overgrown hoof then professional advice and help should be sought. Take care if the animal is heavy in-calf when doing anything which may cause physical stress.

Routine Hoof Trimming

Routine hoof trimming is not generally necessary for animals which are outside for most of the year. For housed animals confined to soft-bedded areas the hooves are bound to overgrow during the winter. Note that some individual animals will be worse than others. Therefore, at turnout in the spring, hoof trimming should be carried out by your vet or a professional hoof trimmer. It is unlikely that you will gain enough experience on a small scale to become an expert hoof trimmer. Even large commercial herds call in the professionals. Leaving overgrown hooves can cause all sorts of strains on the animal, so do have them checked; it causes pain to the animals and affects productivity.

Heavily in-calf cows may limp. The cause may not be the foot but rather a trapped nerve due to the extra bulk the cow is carrying. The problem should solve itself, but if in doubt call the vet.

Worming

The presence of internal and external parasites will add further physical stress which will challenge your animals' overall well-being. Cattle cannot cope with these infestations in a domestic situation without some help. If the internal worm burden gets too high, the animal's physical condition will deteriorate.

The best way to avoid infestation of parasitic worms is to operate a clean grazing system whereby the animals are moved to fresh pasture once within a three week period. This breaks the lifecycle of the parasites. In the absence of clean grazing you will need to treat the animals from time to time with wormers called anthelmintics. Your location and the previous uses of your pasture will affect the frequency and type of wormer you use. It is also important to vary the wormer type as there are resistant strains of worm. Your worming/parasite control regime will be the mainstay of the herd health programme and you should discuss it with your vet at the outset.

Ringworm

Ringworm is a fungal disease affecting the skin. Humans can catch and also be carriers of ringworm. The ringworm fungus can survive in old buildings, utensils, fence posts and so on, seemingly without any time limit, and can be impossible to eradicate unless you scrap the building and put up a new one (highly impractical in most cases). You will need to look out for it.

Symptoms: ringworm is typified by incessant scratching and by round bare patches on the skin on any part of the head or body.

Treatment: there are several proprietary treatments available from your farm supply outlet and fungal spores can eventually be killed by sunshine (ultraviolet light).

Lice

Lice usually affect animals in poor condition, although they do affect healthy stock as well. Housed or confined animals are most susceptible.

Symptoms: lice cause a severe itch. If heavily infested with lice a cow's coat will be damaged, it will be unhappy and its condition will deteriorate.

Treatment: powerful and highly effective injectable and pour-on solutions and powders (which are less effective now as certain ingredients are no longer allowed) are available. Some of these products are combined with wormers (anthelmintics) as well. For those who wish to avoid such products, organically approved louse powders are also available, but these are not very effective.

Mange

Management and nutrition can have a strong influence on the prevalence of this disease. It is caused by a mite which is invisible to the naked eye. It manifests itself by bare patches of coat and flaky skin, with the mites burrowing under the skin. Be aware, however, that not all bare patches automatically mean mange. Cattle, particularly housed ones, do get scruffy coats over the winter, but you will need to be vigilant. Your vet may need to take a skin sample to be analysed under the microscope to confirm that it is mange. The vet will then advise on the correct treatment.

New Forest Disease

This is an infection which occurs when an animal has scratched or damaged its eye in some way.

Symptoms: a weeping, partially closed eye, becoming cloudy and gradually more opaque.

Treatments: a number of treatments are available from your vet. New Forest disease is highly contagious and affected animals should be isolated. However, it is often the case that by the time you notice it, it may already have started to affect others in the herd. Other eye disorders are often erroneously described as New Forest disease. Consult your vet for correct identification of the problem.

Other eye conditions include 'silage eye,' conjunctivitis and chaff-in-the-eye, all with similar symptoms and treatments as described-above. Accurate diagnosis can be made from swab samples to ensure the correct diagnosis and treatment.

Nutritional Disorders

With organic production you are only allowed to provide supplementary vitamins and minerals where there are known deficiencies. Whichever management system you use it is vital that you establish whether or not there are any deficiencies by having your ground tested, as well as by gaining valuable local knowledge from your neighbours. The sooner you know about a problem, the better and you must discuss the best way to deal with the issue with your vet, as dosage levels are critical in some cases.

Molybdenum

High levels of the chemical element molybdenum inhibit the uptake of copper and this has an adverse effect on both growth rates and fertility. Cattle in these areas need a copper supplement added to their diet or given in the form of injections (this is a particular problem in Warwickshire), but this will not solve the problem. By far the most effective treatment is a combination of minerals administered on a slow release basis. Your vet will be able to advise and help you find sustainable long-term solutions.

Selenium

In the New Forest area selenium levels are severely depleted because this trace element has been absorbed by the trees in the forest over hundreds of years. Low selenium levels also have an adverse effect on fertility.

Cobalt

Cobalt is another trace element which is essential for an animal to thrive. Some areas such as Scotland, Northumbria, Devon and North Wales are known to be deficient. Some wormers contain a cobalt supplement.

Salt and Mineral Licks

It is also well known that salt is important to cattle and it is a good idea to provide access to rock salt for most of the year as well as molassed mineral licks to cover all eventualities, particularly if you are out-wintering.

Hypomagnesaemia (magnesium deficiency)

At certain times of the year, particularly autumn and spring, milking cows and cows with calves use up their reserves of magnesium and are then susceptible to hypomagnesaemia, also known as grass sickness or staggers. You can provide high magnesium licks to help minimise the possibility of this happening, particularly if out-wintering cattle.

Note: There is a continuing debate over the possible link with badgers and the spread of bovine tuberculosis. You are advised as a precautionary measure to raise molassed mineral licks to at least 30 inches above the ground to minimise the potential spread of disease as badgers like them too!

Older cattle are more susceptible to hypomagnesaemia as they do not carry more than four or five days' worth of magnesium reserves. It can also affect younger cattle fed on milk alone as the magnesium content of the milk may be variable and is difficult to monitor. This condition may suddenly appear in out-wintered cows, particularly after sudden cold spells or in early spring when their reserves are at their lowest. In spring when the herd is turned out onto pastures which have been fast growing after fertiliser application, the high nitrogen content of the grazing can inhibit the animal's ability to absorb magnesium. This is also the case if it has rained and the grass has grown quickly.

Symptoms: shivering, staggering, falling down, having a fit, kicking and frothing at the mouth.

Prevention: magnesium levels can be raised through careful use of artificial fertilisers. The pasture can be top-dressed (applied to the surface) with magnesium limestone. If there is a major problem on the holding, magnesium oxide can be added to the feed.

Treatment: in an emergency call the vet who will administer the necessary magnesium.

Hypoglycaemia

Better known as Bovine Ketosis/Acetonaemia (reduced blood sugar levels), this may occur when a cow is producing milk at high demand and the level of nutrients she is taking in are insufficient to keep up with the level of production. Swift action is needed.

Symptoms: loss of appetite, constipation and a distinctive sweet smell on the breath. Temperature is normal. Dung is often hard and coated with slime.

Treatment: you should call the vet as major injections are needed to cure this disorder. While you are waiting for the vet to arrive it may help to drench (orally dose) the animal with glucose solution.

Administering a Drench

A plastic cooking oil bottle can be the easiest way to administer a drench. You will need to have the animal restrained (or on a halter at least). Stand by her side behind the head, pass one arm over the neck and reach round and lift up the head by the muzzle. This will result in the mouth being opened. Insert the bottle into the mouth and pour, taking care not to send too much liquid in at once to avoid choking. If the animal is particularly uncooperative you may need to take firm action. You can force the muzzle up by using the nostrils to gain purchase, but you will need to complete the task as quickly as possible as she will like it even less than your first attempt. With really difficult animals, get an assistant to pour as you concentrate on keeping the mouth open. A plastic bottle can also be squeezed to adjust the flow rate to suit the circumstances. You will need to be assertive to dose an animal.

Hypophosphataemia (phosphorus deficiency)

Symptoms: cows in late pregnancy are most at risk. Mild cases are hard to detect, an inability to get up being the most obvious sign. Appetite may be unimpaired.

Prevention and treatment: establish mineral levels on your holding through thorough testing. Provide palatable mineral supplements to counteract any deficiency. Call the vet immediately.

Hypocalcaemia

Also known as Milk Fever (calcium deficiency). This usually affects older cows within 24 hours of calving and, despite all your best efforts to avoid it, milk fever can and does strike. What you must do, however, is act swiftly in your treatment of it.

Symptoms: a loss of appetite, cold ears, shivering, an unsteady weaving walking pattern, constipation, heavy breathing, staggering and eventually going down. The animal may then start tossing herself about. The final stage is coma.

Treatment: as soon as you suspect milk fever, inject 448g (16oz) of calcium solution (first aid kit) under the skin. Massage the site following the injection to disperse the solution. Do this without delay and do not wait for the vet. To prevent pelvic damage hobble (tie together) the back legs to avoid splaying. If you have discovered the animal after it may have been affected for some time, it may be bloated and you may need to take emergency action (see the section on 'ordinary' bloat).

It is essential that you call the vet if any of your animals show the above symptoms as the condition may not be a simple calcium deficiency. Note: the calcium solution you have in your first aid kit will cover other deficiencies such as staggers as well.

It is essential that you seek professional advice and support. If this condition is a recurring problem on your holding your vet will advise on future herd strategy and the longer term nursing of your patient.

Poisoning

Hopefully, through generations of good husbandry, your holding will be free of plants which are dangerous to livestock, but you will still need to be vigilant, particularly if you are reclaiming long disused pasture, woodland or parkland for use with your stock. Below is a list of the most dangerous plants to avoid:

- Yew tree
- Rhododendron
- Acorns
- Ragwort *(an increasing problem due to reduced control measures nationally. Neglected land you are reclaiming may be rife with it. Acquaint yourself with it and remove it on sight, taking it away with you. In dried form it is even more lethal)*
- Laburnum
- Bracken. *(poisoning can unexpectedly affect stock that has lived with the plant for years. It is more common in the spring when the young shoots are more palatable. In upland cattle grazing areas herds are known to live quite happily alongside the bracken, then without warning will consume too much of it and be poisoned. If you have a lot of bracken, seek local advice).*

Do your research and make sure you can identify these plants to avoid a problem in the first place.

Bloat

'Ordinary' bloat is serious, but if treated in time is seldom fatal. It is caused when the animal's main stomach (rumen) fills up with gas. Further study of this ailment is advised. Frothy bloat is far more serious. As the name suggests, the gases form a froth with the contents of the rumen (see below for further discussion of this ailment).

With regard to bloat, prevention is the best form of cure. Before turning animals out on to very lush pasture, provide them with hay or straw to ensure that they have ingested enough fibre and do not have the internal capacity to gorge themselves, particularly if they have been used to poor grazing. Limit the amount of new grazing they have access to by electric fencing and/or limit the time they have access to it. The presence of too much clover increases the risk of bloat considerably. Manure spreading in the winter helps to maintain the correct balance.

Treatment: ask your vet for instruction on emergency actions that you can take if he is unable to attend to your animal quickly. Peanut oil, also known as groundnut oil, and washing soda crystals (in a water solution) can be used as a first aid remedy by drenching as described above (see Hypoglycaemia), but it may be more effective to carefully insert a length of piping down the animal's throat. If a pipe is necessary it is essential that you use a stomach tube designed for the purpose as any other type of tubing could be too rigid and perforate the gullet. Do not be tempted to use thin hosepipe to get the fluid straight to the stomach. Ordinary bloat can be dealt with in a different way by piercing the abdomen on the left-hand side at a specific place with a special tool. You must seek professional help and instruction before attempting this for the first time or you may cause irreparable damage.

Frothy Bloat

Symptoms and causes: frothy bloat can be worse than 'ordinary' bloat in as much as it can be more difficult to save an affected animal. Frothy bloat is more likely to occur if there has been a long dry spell, followed by rain. The pastures will have been semi-dormant due to the dry period, but the rain will have caused the grasses and clovers to grow very quickly. This rapid growth causes the plants to hold high levels of nitrogen and water, but few other minerals and little fibre. The animal will consume it with relish after a winter of dry fodder, but does not produce enough saliva to digest the plant matter properly. A foam forms along with the normal digestive gas, the animal swells, particularly high up on the left-hand side, and it cannot belch or pass wind as the stomach is completely blocked off by the action of the foam, which is made up of minute bubbles.

The area eventually becomes distended and tense. The animal may kick its sides or belly in obvious discomfort, its ears may be back and its breathing increasingly laboured. In the late stages a nose bleed may occur. Eventually the animal will suffocate as the swelling leaves no room for the lungs to work, causing a horrible and painful death. The whole process can be over in an hour or so and if it happens at night you will not even have a chance to intervene.

Remedies and prevention: if you are on old permanent pasture you are at less risk of frothy bloat. However, if you have young grass leys for nitrogen fixing with broad-leafed clover, especially red clover, then there is real danger. If you think your pastures may risk causing frothy bloat, restrict the grazing with electric fencing and provide palatable hay or straw in the field; the cattle will consume it alongside the lush grass to their own benefit. If the animals are housed at night, make sure they come out in the morning full of hay or straw and, if turning cattle out on to fresh spring grass, you can let them have access to anti-bloat licks a few days before These licks can also be provided in the field as well (also dry fodder as above).

An old natural remedy is to pour peanut or linseed oil into the water trough as a preventative measure, but you can never be certain how much each animal will drink if the grass is full of water.

Do not pierce the abdomen in an attempt to cure frothy bloat! It will not help in any way.

If you suspect an animal has frothy bloat it needs to be dosed (drenched) with peanut oil made up of 1 pint (0.57 litres) of peanut (groundnut) oil in some warm water or a quarter of a pound (113g) of washing soda crystals dissolved in hot water and diluted to approximately one pint (0.57 litre) with cold water. You will need help to do this. Do not hold the cow's nose as this will make it more difficult for her. Pass your arm over the nose and calmly and carefully put your hand in the mouth. It is amazing how quickly their stomachs will deflate after drenching. As always call the emergency vet as the animal may need a tube to be inserted into the first stomach to let any gas escape. This should only be attempted by the vet or by someone who is experienced unless it is literally a matter of life or death and help is not available immediately.

Mastitis

Symptoms: inflammation of the udder. You will be able to see that an infected teat looks different, probably swollen. It will feel hotter too. Check each quarter of the udder carefully; it should feel soft and pliable unless engorged with milk. In bad cases the udder feels hard and hot and looks inflamed. To aid diagnosis you could gently try to squeeze some milk out. It may contain clots and look puss-like, a sure sign that you have a problem. Mastitis is more common in milking cows, but it can also be a problem at weaning and particularly during the summer with suckler cows if teats become damaged. Make your cows' udders part of your regular inspections when they are in milk. The cows will become quite used to this as long as you avoid any sudden movements.

Treatment: if you suspect a problem, seek advice from your vet as soon as possible. The condition is very painful for the cow and the calf will be prevented from getting its full ration. Permanent damage can be caused to both the cow and her calf.

Notifiable and Infectious Diseases

A number of diseases are notifiable by law. This means that you must inform your local Animal Health Department if any of them have been diagnosed on your holding. Your vet will advise you of the correct procedures. In addition, in the UK, as part of BSE control measures, the agriculture ministry (Defra) monitors all on-farm deaths of animals greater than 30 months of age. Animals are analysed for the presence of BSE as part of a national monitoring programme. This service is free.

Main notifiable diseases in the UK

- Bluetongue
- Foot and mouth disease
- Anthrax (also zoonose)
- Warble fly infestation
- Bovine Spongiform Encephalopathy (BSE)
- Tuberculosis
- Brucellosis (also zoonose)
- Enzootic bovine leucosis (EBL)
- Johne's disease (also zoonose)

Bluetongue

Until recently Bluetongue was classified as an exotic disease originating in Africa, but already introduced years ago into the Mediterranean countries and the warmer parts of the USA. It is a viral infection that is transmitted by tiny midges called Culicoides. Bluetongue has 24 serotypes, all of which are found on the African continent. Serotype 8, introduced into North-West Europe in 2006, had never before been found anywhere but Africa. Nobody knows the exact route or conditions that brought it to Europe. Either infected midges were brought to Europe in flowers or an animal transporter or the virus came with an infected animal illegally imported from Africa. It was thought that northern species of midges could not become vectors (carriers) of the virus, but once infected our own native midges have ably disproved this

Culicoides have been around for millions of years and can travel great distances on the wind. The pregnant female midge carries the virus after taking blood feeds. The virus multiplies in the midge's blood and then the midge transfers the virus at her next feed.

Cattle tolerate the disease better than sheep, which suffer greatly and are subject to a high mortality rate. If you have sheep on your farm you are far more likely to be alerted by the presence of the disease; in a way they act as sentinels, so it is worth mentioning sheep symptoms here. These include listlessness/lethargy, high temperature, severe lameness, swelling and ulceration in the mouth resulting in drooling, eye and nasal discharges, breathing difficulties, skin haemorrhages and reluctance to rise from the ground when lying down.

Symptoms are less obvious in infected cattle and they recover, but once exposed to the disease it does tend to suppress productivity. They include high temperature, fever, lethargy, sore eyes/conjunctivitis with watery discharge, swelling/ulceration in the mouth, swollen vulva/teats, swelling around the head including the nose/muzzle/eyes/neck and lameness.

Because it is a notifiable disease you must contact the vet at the earliest opportunity if you have even the slightest suspicion of Bluetongue. So be kind to your animals and call the vet, but be aware also that prevention is even better than cure. Your animals are more at risk in warmer months, but these infernal midges have the capacity to function in less favourable periods too, and scientists freely admit that there is much to learn about them.

Although there are various serotypes of the disease, only serotype 8 is active in Northern regions, although both types 1 and 4 are present in Spain, Portugal and Italy. In 2008 type 1 moved from Spain into France, threatening both Belgium and the Netherlands. A vaccine is available for BTV 8, so organise a vaccination programme with your vet as part of your overall herd health plan. Remember that vaccination is vital for both sheep and cattle. It is a very inexpensive option compared to the havoc the disease can wreak. There is no other way to protect your animals from the midges and if your stock do fall victim to the disease, all your vet can do is help reduce any suffering/welfare implications by treating the symptoms. It is not something you can tackle yourself.

Global transport and changing weather patterns and temperatures suggest that bluetongue is not the only 'foreign' disease you need to be aware of. But do not be unduly alarmed. This does not mean your herd is under constant threat and will be exposed, but they are totally dependant on you, their keeper, being well informed. You can find lots more impartial and reliable information about this and other threats by visiting www.ela-europe.org

Zoonoses

These are animal diseases that can be transferred to humans. Some of the notifiable diseases which are also transmissible to humans have been eradicated in the UK, for instance the last case of brucellosis confirmed in the UK was in 1993. It is, however, incumbent upon you as a responsible keeper to be aware of these particularly dangerous disease threats. Rather than include a detailed doomsday list here, you will find more detailed information at the Defra website at www.defra.gov.uk/ani-malh for up-to-date information. On a global level, wherever you are, go to the website for the World Organisation for Animal Health at www.oie.int.

E. coli

A generally misunderstood threat to you, your family and most likely any visitors to your farm, is E. coli. There are harmful strains of this otherwise benign bacteria which cause potentially severe stomach upsets and illness and so it must be taken seriously. Outbreaks of E. coli poisoning regularly make the news and in a rather alarmist fashion. This has had the unfortunate and unnecessary effect of schools ending visits to open farms. A theory amongst livestock keepers is that visitors who do not have regular contact with animals are less resistant if exposed to E. coli bacteria.

Prevention is simple – sensible hygiene precautions must be observed at all times and this includes you! If you have touched the animals, have been mucking out, or have been sprayed with slurry or urine if you were in the wrong place at the wrong time, then wash your hands and any other part of you that has been af-

fected as soon as is practical. Keep your hands away from your mouth. As far as farm visits in the UK are concerned your local Health and Safety Authority will have their own rules and guidelines for organised visits which you must implement. They will include simple things like the availability of washing facilities, wet wipes etc.

Notifiable Diseases

BSE (Bovine Spongiform Encephalopathy)

Symptoms: muscle tremors, aggression, staggering and loss of use of the back legs. This is not to be confused with hypomagnesaemia and other conditions with similar symptoms as you are more likely to come across these latter ailments.

Action: contact your vet immediately on seeing the above symptoms. This is a notifiable disease. In the UK when acquiring stock you can find out the BSE history of the source farm from Defra.

Foot and Mouth Disease

Symptoms: affected milking animals show a sudden drop in milk production together with blisters in the mouth, slobbering, sucking, high temperature, discomfort, pain when walking and blisters between the claws.

Action: report these symptoms to your vet immediately as this is an extremely contagious, legally notifiable disease.

Tuberculosis and Brucellosis

Your herd will be tested for TB and brucellosis at the expense of Defra once every two years.

Herd tests are co-ordinated and carried out by your vet. You do need to be aware that some parts of the country are more badly affected than others and you should do all you can to minimise the potential risks to your herd. Send for information from Defra. Tuberculosis and brucellosis are both notifiable diseases. If buying cattle from a known TB 'hotspot' have the animals tested before delivery. It makes no sense to bring infected animals to a clean area.

TB is probably the greatest health threat of all to cattle in the UK. Study the issues carefully and stay informed. In the UK the debate currently rages on about the causes and methods of transmission and whether or not badgers are involved in the transmission.

Other Ailments and Diseases

The following is a list of some of the other ailments and diseases you should be aware of: husk, fog fever, choke; big leg, black leg, redwater (a tick-borne disease found in particular in Wales, Scotland, South West England, Devon, Dorset and Northern England), tetanus, leptospirosis, blaine, photosensitisation, wooden tongue, viral pneumonia, IBR, catarrhal fever, bovine viral diarrhoea, salmonellosis, liver fluke infection and mud fever. This is not a complete list and does not include tropical diseases for readers in those areas.

Administering Medicines

Keep first aid equipment to hand to enable you to give simple medication without calling the vet. Instructions for different medicines are on the bottle or pack. Read them carefully to be sure you are choosing the right option and dose and ask your vet to provide you with the medicines you should have to hand which cannot be purchased from your agricultural merchant. Your vet will also give you instruc-tion on how to give basic injections and how to dose animals orally (drenching). There are three types of basic injection:

1. Subcutaneous: the needle slides sideways under the skin but does not pierce the muscle. The medicine rests under the skin and is absorbed slowly. This is the least painful injection for the animal unless you are administering a solution which stings.
2. Intramuscular: the medicine is injected straight into a muscle. Your vet will demonstrate the best method.
3. Intravenous: the needle is placed into a vein. This is a potentially life-threatening procedure if attempted by the inexperienced. On no account attempt intravenous injections without having had the proper training.

In addition you should keep the following:
- Antibiotic spray (for wounds, sore hooves, navel dressing)
- Thermometer (digital ones are easy to read and are not too expensive)
- Scour (diarrhoea) formula (particularly if calf rearing)
- Colostrum substitute
- Liquid iodine (for wounds and navel dressing)
- Disinfectant (for washing the operative's or vet's hands as well as for cleaning surfaces or instruments)
- Magnesium and calcium solutions (for staggers - always keep this in stock and make sure it is within its use by date. If you find yourself in an emergency and do not have any to hand you will probably be too late)
- Obstetric gel (for assisted calvings)
- 16 gauge x 1 inch disposable needles
- Disposable syringes, mostly 20ml but also a few 50ml
- 50ml dosing (drenching) syringes
- Bandage and wound dressings
- Calving ropes
- Stomach tube kit
- Weak calf reviver

DIAGNOSTIC GUIDE TO CATTLE AILMENTS AND TREATMENT		
Signs of Disease	Causes	Treatment and Prevention
HEAD AND FACE		
Nasal discharge.	Pneumonia due to bacterial, viral or parasitic infection. Bluetongue (NB. notifiable disease).	Antibiotic for bacterial infection. Wormers for parasitic infection. If indoors, check ventilation. Vaccinate where appropriate.
Ulcers on lips, mouth and tongue.	Mucosal disease or Foot and Mouth disease (NB. notifiable disease). Malignant catarrh.	These are all due to virus infection. Antibiotic will control secondary bacterial infection. Control is through vaccination, cleaning and disinfection and, with Foot and Mouth in the UK, slaugher policy.
Salivation and drooling from mouth.	Ulcers (see above). Infection in tongue or mouth (lumpy jaw or wooden tongue). Obstruction in mouth or gullet eg. choking due to potato or similar, or tumour.	Antibiotic for any general infection. Potassium iodide orally or sodium iodide intravenously. Remove foreign body if appropriate. In case of tumour slaughter on welfare grounds.
Swelling of lips and tongue - tongue has blue appearance.	Bluetongue (NB. notifiable disease), viral disease.	Vaccinate for Bluetongue.
Loss of hair from face and muzzle.	Photosensitisation, but only outdoors.	Move indoors, corticosteroids and antihistamines.
Loss of hair with scabs on face.	Ringworm (NB. infectious to people).	Topical antifungal agents.
EYES		
Discharge from both eyes.	Contagious infection eg. New Forest Disease or symptom of more general infection eg. malignant catarrhal fever or muscosal disease.	Topical eye treatment. General infection needs antibiotic, good nursing care and electrolytes.
Discharge from one eye.	Possible foreign body eg. hay seed/straw. May also be unilateral infection.	Remove foreign body. Apply topical antibiotic.
Swollen eye lids.	Allergic reaction.	Antihistamines or corticosteroids.
Eyes dull and lifeless.	General debility due to disease or deficiency.	Check for other symptoms. Treat general symptoms.
Blindness.	Cataracts. Pus or blood in eye due to trauma or infection. Lead poisoning. Vitamin deficiencies eg. vitamin A or thiamine.	Nothing practical can be done. Some traumatic damage will repair. Calcium versenate. Give vitamins. Antibiotic eye cream.
Yellow with colour in white of the eye.	Jaundice due to infection of liver or liver damage due to poisoning eg. ragwort or tumour. Redwater Fever (Babesiosis).	Antibiotic and vitamins. Good nursing and carbohydrate diet. Endoparasite treatment. Eradicate ticks from pasture.

Signs of Disease	Causes	Treatment and Prevention
EYES CONTINUED		
Mucosa of eye - pale or white.	Anaemia due to worms or deficient diet. Poisoning eg. bracken or brassica. Redwater Fever due to Babesia infection.	Improve diet/give iron. Deworm with anthelmintic. Check for cobalt or copper deficiency. Remove source of poison. Use endoparasiticide for Babesia infection. Eradicate ticks from pasture.
Mucosa of eye - dark and congested.	Circulatory problem as part of a more generalised disease eg. Pneumonia.	Treat general disease/check for other symptoms. Seek veterinary help.
Eyes sunk into eye sockets.	Dehydration usually as the result of scouring.	Check for cause of scour. Electrolytes and fluid replacement/drip may be required. Antibiotic if infection is present.
EARS		
One or both ears swollen.	Abscess or blood blister due to badly applied ear tag or other injury.	Drain abscess/leave haematoma. May require topical antibiotic treatment.
One ear drooping/pus discharging.	Infection eg. Listeriosis.	Antibiotic eg. oxytetracycline for Listeria infection. Make better silage.
SKIN AND HAIR		
Coat colour changes without hair loss.	Copper/zinc (rare) cobalt/manganese deficiency.	Blood samples required to confirm diagnosis before treatment of deficiency. Anthelmintic for worms.
Loss of coat without itch.	Parasitic gastroenteritis (gut worms). Rain scald due to Dermatophilus infection.	Antibiotics eg. oxytetracycline and penicillin/streptomycin. Improve housing conditions. Treat for worms if appropriate.
Loss of hair with round, raised crusty lesions.	Ringworm (NB.infectious to people).	Topical antifungal agents.
Loss of hair with itching.	Ectoparasites eg. lice or mange mites.	Skin scrapings may be required to confirm mange infection. Louse powders and mange washes. Pour on preparations eg. Ivermectin.
Raised sore areas in unpigmented part of coat.	Photosensitisation due to sunlight. Animal often becomes sensitive by eating plants such as St. John's Wort or rape.	House indoors, treat with antihistamines, corticosteroids and sun blocking creams. Remove offending plants.
Soft swellings on back.	Warble fly (now eradicated in the UK but notifiable if discovered).	Ectoparasitical preparations (pour on and injectable).

The Smallholder's Guide to Animal Ailments

Signs of Disease	Causes	Treatment and Prevention
BREATHING		
Rapid breathing.	Pneumonia due to viral, bacterial or parasitic infection eg. lungworm. Stress as the result of pain, overheating or exercise. Heart disease or clot in main vein to heart. Bluetongue (NB. notifiable disease). Fog Fever (see below).	Antibiotic and anti-inflammatory drugs. Anthelmintic for lungworm. Vaccine for prevention. Get expert to check ventilation. Remove source of stress. Casualty slaughter may be the only solution. No effective treatment. Vaccinate. Corticosteroids.
Shallow breathing.	Asleep or Hypocalcaemia if recumbent (milk fever). Terminal stage of any illness.	Check for other symptoms. Calcium injection usually effective (subcutaneous or intravenous).
Coughing.	Symptom of respiratory disease eg. Pneumonia due to virus, bacteria or lungworm. Foreign material in windpipe due to incorrect dosing or drenching. Fog Fever due to intoxication with L-tryptophan. Occurs in autumn on lush grazing.	Antibiotic/anti-inflammatory and mucolytic drugs. Anthelmintic for lungworm. Inhalation Pneumonia. Little can be done apart from antibiotic for infection. Corticosteroids and anti-inflammatory drugs may help. Remove cattle from lush grazing.
TEMPERATURE (normal range is 101.5-102.5°F)		
Raised.	Usually means animal has infection, but may be the result of pain or stress.	Antibiotic required for most infections. Check for other symptoms. Pain killers may be necessary. If high temperature persists, get advice.
Lowered.	Check reading again, may be incorrect technique/hypothermia or terminally ill.	If correct, raise body temperature with heat lamps or equivalent. It needs diagnosis . Get advice.
Sweating.	See above for raised temperature.	See above for raised temperature.
Shivering.	See above for lowered temperature.	See above for lowered temperature.
DUNG		
Constipation.	Indigestion and reduced feed intake. Acetonaemia/Ketosis.	Check diet and look for other symptoms. Corticosteroids, intravenous glucose, vitamins, propylene glycol.

Signs of Disease	Causes	Treatment and Prevention
DUNG CONTINUED		
Scouring.	Nutritional eg. too much rich grass.	Feed hay before turning out.
	Bacterial infection eg. Johne's Disease (NB. notifiable in N. Ireland).	Antibiotic, but no treatment for Johne's Disease.
	Virus infection eg. Mucosal disease/ malignant catarrhal fever/ infectious Bovine Rhino-tracheitis.	Antibiotic to cover secondary infection, fluid and supportive therapy.
	Parasites eg. worms/fluke/coccidia.	Anthelmintic.
	Plant or other poisoning.	Find and remove source of poison and treat symptoms.
Scouring with blood.	Salmonella (NB. infectious to people). Coccidiosis. Vibrionic (Campylobacter) scour.	Antibiotic/fluid therapy/good nursing. Oral antibiotic. All above require good hygienic precautions. Some types of salmonella can be vaccinated against.
	Cancer.	Slaughter on welfare grounds.
Abdominal distension with fluid.	Pregnant.	Get vet to confirm.
	Heart disease.	Poor prognosis.
	Peritonitis.	May respond to antibiotic, but generally poor outlook.
Abdominal distension, left side abdomen. ie. bloat.	Gas not being belched from rumen.	Remove foreign body or push it down into rumen.
	Due to obstruction eg. potato or failure in nervous mechanism which allows belching or frothy bloat where gas and fluid are mixed as froth.	Pass stomach tube to relieve simple bloat. Drench with cooking oil or linseed oil to relieve frothy bloat. Chronic cases can be cured by a vet making a permanent fistula.
	Impaction as the result of a high fibre diet.	Check diet in all above cases.
Bloat with distension on both sides of abdomen.	Severe bloat, animal will be near to death.	May require emergency trocarisation. Get the vet as soon as possible.

Signs of Disease	Causes	Treatment and Prevention
URINE		
Urinary retention or inability to pass urine ie.Urolithiasis.	Calculi in urethra may cause partial or total blockage.	Muscle relaxant drug may be all that is required in cases of partial blockage. Complete blockage requires immediate attention and often surgery. See vet urgently.
	Due to dietary imbalance of mineral, usually magnesium.	Check diet/add salt to diet as prevention.
Blood in urine.	Cystitis, bacterial infection eg. clostridial or leptospiral infection (NB. Leptospirosis infectious to people).	Vaccine can be used to prevent clostridial or leptospiral infection.
	Kidney infection.	Antibiotic for routine infection in bladder and kidney.
	Brassica/bracken poisoning. Nitrite poisoning.	Antibiotic and drip to treat bracken cases/ same for brassica cases plus vitamins and iron. Remove source of poison. Methylene blue solution for nitrite cases.
	Red Water Fever, result of infection with Babesia.	Endoparasiticides/blood may be required/ eradicate ticks from pasture.
Pain in abdomen; seen as lying down and getting up frequently, teeth grinding and kicking while lying down.	Colic due to intestinal inflammation or obstruction. Urolithiasis (see above).	Muscle relaxant and pain killing drugs may be all that is required. Severe blockages eg. twisted bowel or Urolithiasis require surgery.
	Peritonitis.	Antibiotic, poor outlook.
	Lead poisoning.	Calcium versenate.
	Foreign body in rumen penetrating into liver and chest.	Surgery to retrieve foreign material/successful if carried out early.
Swelling at navel.	Rupture.	Surgery rarely indicated. Usually better, unless animal is very valuable, to go for economic slaughter.
Fluid swelling along from udder.	Udder Oedema if just prior to, or after calving.	No treatment usually indicated. Swelling will go after a few days.
Fluid along brisket and abdomen.	Heart failure which may be primary or due to foreign body penetration from abdomen.	Diuretics may be helpful in minor cases, but seldom practical.

Signs of Disease	Causes	Treatment and Prevention
INFERTILITY - FEMALE		
Failure to come into season.	Pregnant or failure to detect season or low body weight or deficiency disease eg. copper, manganese. Infection eg. Brucellosis (NB. notifiable disease and infectious to people). Ovarian problems eg. persistent corpus luteum. Congenital eg. freemartinism.	Vet required to check for any possible pregnancy. All other conditions require correct diagnosis before vet can apply correct treatment. Cull from herd.
Abortion.	Infection eg. Brucellosis and Leptospirosis (NB. Brucellosis notifiable disease, both infectious to people). Any disease which causes a rise in temperature eg. virus or bacteria. Fungal infection. Clumsy management and poor handling.	In case of Brucellosis cull from herd. For leptospiral infection use antibiotic and can vaccinate. Investigate cause of abortion by blood test and swabs before attempting treatment. Good hygiene is essential at all times and isolate the cow until the cause of abortion is known.
Vaginal discharge- clear/with or without blood stain.	If pregnant may be about to give birth. Slight discharge can be apparent when in season.	Get experienced help to check. If in season will display behavioural signs.
Purulent smelly discharge with or without afterbirth being retained.	Primary infection in genital tract or due to retained afterbirth, which may be hanging from vulva.	Antibiotic either by injection or by inserting pessaries or by irrigation. Remove afterbirth.
INFERTILITY - MALE		
	Specific infection eg. Brucellosis (NB. notifiable disease). Deficiency disease eg. iodine, manganese or vitamin A. Orthopaedic problems eg. sore back, legs or pelvis.	Infertility difficult to diagnose. Will require sperm counts and blood tests. Get vet to check and treat any lameness.
MASTITIS		
Blood in milk.	Can be quite normal just after calving.	No treatment required. Will resolve in a day or two.
Milk very thick after calving.	Colostrum.	Normal, no treatment required.
Clots in milk.	Mild form of Mastitis due to infection by Streptococcus.	Antibiotic. Check bacterial sensitivity before treatment. Management may be at fault.
Watery milk.	Possible Coliform Mastitis.	Antibiotic as above.
Udder very hot and cow ill.	Severe Mastitis possible. Corynebacterium Pyogenes or summer Mastitis.	Antibiotic both in the udder and by injection. May require emergency vet treatment to save life.
Milk drop.	Leptospiral (NB. infectious to people) or Mycoplasma infection. Mastitis.	Investigate before treatment with antibiotic.

Signs of Disease	Causes	Treatment and Prevention
MASTITIS		
Teat abnormalities.	Virus infection eg. herpes or cow pox. Chapped or eroded teat ends.	Bland ointments/udder cream. Check milking machine and management.
LAMENESS		
Feet.	Interdigital infection eg. foul in the foot or puncture wound.	Antibiotics. May need to pare away the infected part.
	Septic arthritis in the foot joint.	Surgery may be required. See vet.
	Laminitis due to overeating.	Analgesics, warm water bathing to improve circulation. Methionine in diet may be helpful.
	Virus infection ie. Foot and Mouth disease (NB. notifiable disease).	Call vet.
	Bluetongue (NB. notifiable disease).	Call vet. No effective treatment. Vaccinate.
Limbs.	Injury eg. fracture, nerve damage, puncture wounds and sprains.	All but most minor need vet attention. Treat symptoms.
	Arthritis.	Analgesics and anti-inflammatory drugs. Antibiotic.
	Joint infections. Blackleg due to clostridial infection of the muscle.	High dose of antibiotic and clostridial antiserum. Poor prognosis. Good vaccine available.
BEHAVIOUR		
Loss of appetite.	Any factor which causes a rise in temperature.	Check for other symptoms. Look in mouth for sores and blisters.
	Pain.	Fluids, glucose, corticosteroids.
	Acetonaemia due to negative energy balance (poor feeding management).	Improve feeding management.
	Acidosis due to gorging on carbohydrate.	Electrolytes, multivitamins, antihistamines.
	Indigestion due to dysfunction of the vagus nerve.	Poor prognosis. Treat symptoms, stomach drenches, stimulants and good nursing.

Signs of Disease	Causes	Treatment and Prevention
BEHAVIOUR CONTINUED		
Nervous signs eg. blindness, head pressing, staggering gait, excitement.	Hypomagnesaemia (low blood magnesium).	Magnesium sulphate (subcutaneous injection) and sedation.
	Milk fever (low blood calcium).	Calcium borogluconate (intravenous or subcutaneous injection).
	Lead poisoning, usually from licking old paint.	Calcium versenate injection - get the vet. Remove source of old paint.
	Nervous signs of acetonaemia.	See above.
	Listeriosis.	Antibiotic.
	Louping ill due to virus infection.	No specific treatment. Remove bracken as a source of tick. Vaccine is available.
Nervous signs eg. walking in a circle.	Gid (parasitic tapeworm cyst on brain) or brain abscess, tumour or haemorrhage.	Surgical removal of cyst. Worm dogs as they carry the tapeworm. Slaughter on welfare grounds may be necessary.
Nervous signs eg. any change in normal behaviour.	Bovine Spongiform Encephalopathy (BSE) (NB. notifiable disease).	Slaughter policy.
Nervous signs eg. convulsions and collapse.	Hypomagnesaemia (see above).	See above.
	Terminal signs of any nervous disease.	Euthanasia may be required on welfare grounds.
RECUMBENCY		
Unable to stand and walk.	Milk fever due to low blood calcium levels.	Calcium borogluconate by subcutaneous or intravenous injection.
	Downer cow syndrome/often follows milk fever/ nerve and muscle damage.	Good nursing, stimulants, sling or lift patient with air bags.
	Physical injury.	Good nursing, treat symptomatically.
	Terminal stages of any fatal illness.	May require euthanasia on welfare grounds.
SUDDEN DEATH		
Without prior warning.	Anthrax (NB. notifiable disease and infectious to people).	All sudden deaths must be checked by law. Get vet.
	Bloat (see above). Plant poisoning eg. yew, laburnum.	Never leave hedge or tree clippings where an animal can reach them.
	Blackleg. Hypomagnesaemia.	Effective vaccines are available. Prevent with supplements or bolus.
	Lightning strike. Electrocution.	Scorch marks may be seen on the skin. Check wiring!

DIAGNOSTIC GUIDE TO CALF AILMENTS AND TREATMENT

Signs of Disease	Causes	Treatment and Prevention
HEAD AND FACE		
Nasal discharge.	Pneumonia/bacteria/virus/parasites.	Antibiotics for infection, wormers for lung-worm. Check ventilation. Vaccinate where appropriate.
Ulcers on lips and mouth.	Pox virus/mucosal disease/Foot and Mouth disease (NB. notifiable disease)/ malignant cararrhal fever.	Antibiotic for secondary infection. Call vet if Foot and Mouth is suspected.
Salivation and drooling from mouth.	Ulcers (see above). Infection in tongue or mouth eg. calf Diphtheria. Obstruction in mouth or gullet.	Antibiotics for an infection. Remove foreign body, if appropriate.
Loss of hair from face/muzzzle.	Photosensitisation but only outdoors. Vitamin A deficiency in milk fed calves.	Move indoors, steroids and antihistamines. Give vitamins until calf is eating creep feed.
Loss of hair with scabs on face.	Ringworm (NB infectious to people).	Topical antifungal agents.
Loss of hair around mouth.	Milk scald due to bucket feeding.	Will resolve when bucket feeding stops.
EYES		
Discharge from both eyes.	Contagious infection eg. New Forest disease or symptom of more general infection eg Pneumonia.	Treat with antibiotic in eyes or if more general by injection.
Discharge from one eye.	Possible foreign body eg. hay seed. Turned in eye lid.	Remove. Minor operation required.
Swollen eye lids.	Allergic reaction.	Antihistamines or corticosteroids.
Eyes dull and lifeless.	Part of general disease eg. Pneumonia or scours.	Treat general symptoms.
Blindness.	Congenital cataracts. Lead poisoning. Vitamin deficiency eg. vitamin A or thiamine. Infection.	Nothing can be done. Calcium versenate. Give vitamins. Antibiotics.
Yellow colour in white of eye.	Jaundice due to liver disease or liver damage.	Antibiotics and vitamins. High carbohydrate diet.
Mucosa of eye - pale or white.	Anaemia due to worms or deficient diet.	Improve diet/give iron/kill worms with anthelmintic.
Mucosa of eye - dark and congested.	Circulation problem as part of a more general disease eg Pneumonia.	Treat general disease. See vet.
Eyes sunk into sockets.	Dehydration, usually caused by scouring.	Electrolytes as fluid replacers/antibiotics if infection present.

Signs of Disease	Causes	Treatment and Prevention
EARS		
One or both ears swollen.	Abscess or blood blister due to badly applied ear tag or injury.	Drain abscess/leave haematoma/vet to decide treatment.
One ear drooping/pus discharging.	Infection/possible Listeriosis (NB. infectious to people).	Antibiotics.
SKIN AND HAIR		
Coat colour changes without hair loss.	Copper/zinc (rare) cobalt/maganese deficiency. Parasitic gastroenteritis (gut worms).	Blood samples required for diagnosis before treatment for deficiencies. Anthelmintic for worms.
Loss of coat without itching.	Rain scald due to Dermatophilus infection.	Antibacterial and improve housing conditions.
Loss of coat with round, raised crusty lesions.	Ringworm (NB. infectious to people).	Topical antifungal agent .
Loss of coat with itching.	Ectoparasites eg. lice or mange mites.	Louse powders/mange washes/pour on preparations eg. Ivermectin.
Raised sore areas in unpigmented part of coat.	Photosensitisation due to sunlight. Animal has been sensitised by eating plants such as St. John's Wort or rape.	House indoors/treat with antihistamines, corticosteroids and sun blocking creams.
Growths on skin surface.	Warts or angleberries.	Most warts resolve spontaneously. Autogenous vaccine can be made for severe lesions. Surgery may be required. See vet.
BREATHING		
Rapid breathing.	Pneumonia due to virus, bacteria or parasites eg. lungworm. Stress due to pain or overheating or exercise.	Antibiotics and anti-inflammatory drugs. Anthelmintic for lungworm. Vaccinate to prevent. Get expert to check environment. Remove source of stress.
Shallow breathing.	Asleep or in terminal stage of illness.	No action. Check for other symptoms. Call vet.
Coughing.	Respiratory disease eg. Pneumonia due to bacteria/virus or parasite. Foreign material in windpipe due to bad drenching or dosing.	Antibiotics, anti-inflammatory agents and mucolytics. See vet. Remove foreign body if possible. Antibiotics for secondary infection.
TEMPERATURE (normal range is 101.5-102.5°F)		
Raised.	Usually means infection but may be the result of stress or pain.	Antibiotic for infection/remove source of stress. Analgesics for pain. See vet.
Lowered.	Check again. Incorrect technique or hypothermia or terminally ill.	If correct, raise body temperature with heat lamps or equivalent. Get advice.
Sweating.	See above for raised temperature.	See above for raised temperature.
Shivering.	See above for lowered temperature.	See above for lowered temperature.

Signs of Disease	Causes	Treatment and Prevention
DUNG		
Constipation.	Rarely a problem.	Check diet.
Scouring.	Milk scour due to overfeeding.	Stop or reduce milk intake and give electrolytes.
	Bacterial infection eg E. coli or Salmonella (NB. Infectious to people).	Antibiotics for bacterial infections/good general nursing care -keep clean and warm.
	Virus or coccidial infection.	Vaccines may help control virus infections.
	Consider possible worm infestation if out at grass.	Anthelmintic to get rid of worm burden.
Scouring with blood.	Salmonella infection likely if very depressed (NB. infectious to people).	Antibiotics and a high standard of nursing care is required.
	Coccidiosis.	Coccidiostat normally very effective.
Bloat ie. abdominal distension of the left side of abdomen.	Gas not being belched from rumen. Due either to obstruction in the gullet or failure in the mechanism to allow belching or frothy bloat where gas and fluid are mixed as a froth.	Remove foreign body from gullet. Pass stomach tube to relieve simple bloat. Drench with linseed oil or cooking oil to relieve frothy bloat. Check diet in all cases.
Bloat with distention on both sides of abdomen.	Severe bloat, animal will be close to death.	May require emergency trocarisation. Get the vet as soon as possible.
URINE		
Urinary retention or blockage ie. Urolithiasis.	Calculi in urethra may cause partial or total blockage. Cause is usually dietary imbalance of mineral, usually magnesium.	Muscle relaxant drug may be all that is required in cases of partial blockage. Surgery often necessary. Call vet urgently. For control add salt to diet.
Blood in urine.	Infection eg. clostridial or acute leptospiral disease (NB. infectious to people) or brassica poisoning eg. kale.	High doses of antibiotic required for infection. Stop feeding brassica/vitamin and iron injections. Severe cases may require blood transfusions.
Pain in abdomen; seen as lying down and getting up frequently, teeth grinding and kicking while lying down.	Colic due to intestinal inflammation or obstruction.	Muscle relaxant drugs may be all that is required. Severe blockage eg. twisted bowel or Urolithiasis require surgery.
	Urolithiasis (see above).	
	Peritonitis.	Antibiotics, poor outlook.
	Lead poisoning.	Calcium versenate. Get the vet.

Signs of Disease	Causes	Treatment and Prevention
Swelling at the navel.	Rupture.	No action if small. Surgery indicated if swelling is large.
	Abscess at navel due to infection getting in at birth.	Antibiotic at high doses. May be difficult to clear.
Fluid lower belly.	Calculi in the urethra blocking the flow of urine.	Surgery almost always the only treatment. See vet.
LAMENESS		
Feet.	Interdigital infection eg. foul in the foot or puncture wound.	Antibiotics and may need to pare away the infected part.
	Laminitis due to overfeeding.	Analgesics, warm water bathing to improve circulation. Methionine in the diet.
	Virus infection eg. Foot and Mouth disease (NB. notifiable disease).	Call the vet.
Limbs.	Injury eg. fracture, nerve damage, puncture wound, joint ill ie. infection.	All but the most minor need vet attention. Treat symptoms. Antibiotics as early as possible.
	Rickets.	Calcium and vitamin D.
	If stiff and unable to rise consider vitamin E deficiency.	Vitamin E injections.
BEHAVIOUR		
Loss of appetite.	Rise in temperature. Pain.	Check for other symptoms; look in mouth for sores.
Nervous signs eg. walking in circles or head pressing.	Cerebrocortical necrosis (CCN) ie. thiamine deficiency. Lead poisoning, usually from licking old paint. Infection eg. Listeriosis (NB. infectious to people) causing microabscesses in brain. Gid (tapeworm or cyst on brain) or brain abscess, brain haemorrhage or brain tumour.	Inject thiamine. Control with roughage in diet and brewers grains. Calcium versenate injection and get rid of source. Antibiotic. Silage may be the source. Surgical removal of cyst. Worm dogs as they carry the tapeworm. Slaughter on welfare grounds may be necessary.
Nervous signs eg. convulsions.	Hypomagnesaemia due to a drop in blood magnesium. Terminal signs of any nervous disease.	Injections of magnesium with or without calcium. Sedative. Euthanasia may be required on welfare grounds.
SUDDEN DEATH		
Without prior warning.	Anthrax (NB.notifiable disease and infectious to people) Bloat (see above). Poisoning. Hypomagnesmia. Lightning strike or electrocution.	Get the vet to check in all cases by doing a post-mortem when necessary. Don't leave hedge or tree clippings where animals can reach them. Prevent with supplements or bolus. Check for scorch marks on skin. Get a qualified person to check wiring.

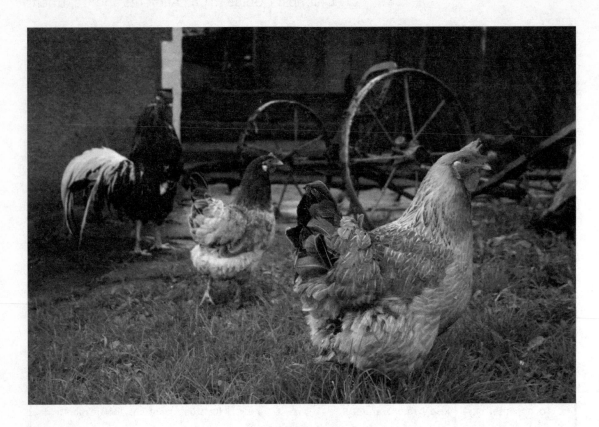

Chapter Two

CHICKEN DISEASES

By Paul Peacock

There are some important jobs a poultry keeper must be sure of. They are fundamental to the way you cope with keeping poultry. More than anything, other than bee-keeping, keeping poultry is a matter of good practice, careful routine and confidence. Being confident, knowing you have an appropriate plan for all eventualities – even if this means getting help elsewhere, is the best foundation for good poultry keeping.

The first important thing you should do with your chickens is to find a vet who knows something about them! You don't want to be paying out thirty pounds a visit while the vet scratches his head and looks it up in a book. Your local poultry club will have a list of the best vets for poultry in your area.

Set yourself the routine of providing your hens with a substrate that you can change. This is usually fresh pasture, but if you have poultry in a small garden this might not be possible. You can provide a pit filled with wood chips or bark which you can remove and compost. Providing fresh pasture or places for them to walk and scratch about every three months keeps the burden of worms at bay. Worms are one of the biggest problems in the chicken world.

Learn too how to kill a chicken in the correct manner so that its death is painless. It is frequently the best way of treating the animal with humane kindness rather than letting it suffer. In reality it is difficult to learn this from a book and you are best being taught. Sadly many people do the job incorrectly. It is perhaps strange starting a chapter on hen veterinary welfare with instructions on how to kill a bird, but it is a basic and important part of our care for our livestock. The following procedure is how you should kill a chicken.

Prepare your animals for this final act by handling them regularly; this way they will not be distressed when you approach.
Pick them up gently but firmly and hold both legs in a firm grip with one hand.
Hold the head between the middle fingers of the other hand so that the back of the head rests in your palm.
Push down on the head and twist and you should feel the bones break and the animal will begin to flap violently. This will stop very quickly and the bird will be dead.
Hold the bird upside down and cut the neck with a knife.

In my own opinion and that of Compassion in World Farming, you should not use clamps or neck dislocators which hurt the bird or cause it distress. Similarly, the 'killing cone' favoured in the US can increase the anxiety experienced by a bird.

Red Mite

There are a number of mites your hens will collect almost out of thin air and unless you keep them under control they will make your animal very uncomfortable at best or, at worst, kill it.

Red mite is your introduction to poultry diseases. For the new poultry keeper not used to red mite they are entirely unexpected. One minute your hens are fine, then all of a sudden they get a little scaly leg, which in itself seems very minor. Then you notice the perch is covered with red mites, all huddled together in the shade.

These tiny red things are full of chicken's blood and move slowly away from the light in a crepuscular fashion: suddenly, for the first time, you understand that animals can be quite unpleasant.

Red mites have 8 legs and no body divisions. Like spiders they are arachnids. They live away from the animal during the day, hiding in crevices in huts, in nest boxes or anywhere they can find shade. During the night they march out like a small army onto the legs of the bird to pierce the skin and drink its blood.

Treatment

The best treatment for red mite is to keep them down to the minimum levels by attacking them where they spend the day. Clean out the hut and give it a jet wash as often as you can. You can also buy powders and sprays to treat the birds, but it is little use treating them if you are not going to treat the hut too. Pyrethroids, organophosphates, carbamates, citrus extracts, vegetable/sunflower oil and mineral-based products (both liquids and dusts) have been used to control red mite in the environment. Covering with sunflower oil will also slow down their return. Make sure you get into the nest boxes. These mites can live for six months on a single belly full of blood, so you will have to be on your guard!

Northern Fowl Mite

Northern fowl mite stay on the birds all the time and so have a more devastating effect. You should look for listless or irritated birds. They will have a loss of condition, pale combs and wattles, spots of blood on the eggs and the number of eggs produced will begin to drop. They are more difficult to spot than red mite.

The mites also carry other problems such as fowl cholera and, as the birds become more heavily infested, they cannot replace the lost blood quickly enough, leading to anaemia and other immunological problems, at which point they can go down with almost anything.

Treatment

Recognising northern fowl mite is a rotten task. You will find mites near the neck and around the vent, together with their with eggs and faeces. The feathers will be stained dark, and I cannot stand them running onto my hand. (Yes, I know I'm squeamish!).

For northern fowl mite it is essential to apply approved insecticides to affected birds as there is little else available. You will need to ensure the birds are treated each fortnight until they are gone, and you must ensure that the appropriate set aside periods are adhered to before any birds are killed for meat. There are, however, lots of treatments available where the eggs have no set aside.

Mite levels in the flock may never come down to zero, and you shouldn't treat and treat until you have removed the last mite. You should, however, maintain a regular treatment for mites every month or so. If you are vigilant you should have happy hens.

Lice

Lice can be detected like mites, but are usually somewhat larger. There are three major ones; the poultry louse, the scaly leg louse and the depluming louse.

The poultry louse is found at the vent and the neck and is flattish and yellowish. Its scratching of the skin, its excrement and its general presence irritate the bird no end. They lay their eggs at the base of the feathers and the larvae eat the skin scales as they emerge.

The scaly leg louse gets under the scales of the bird's legs and, in bad cases, the skin forms calluses which irritate the bird.

The depluming louse bothers the bird so much that she will actually pull out her feathers in order to gain some respite.

Treatment is by a regular dusting with louse powder. Some people coat the legs with oils or even dip them in alcohol. The treatment of choice, louse powder, works very well and there are no withdrawal times for either meat or eggs.

Worms

Intestinal Roundworms are common. Birds become droopy and have diarrhoea, with worms clearly visible in the droppings. These are not to be confused with fungal roundworm in humans which isn't a worm at all.

Caecal Worms come from the soil. Chickens ingest them and in certain circumstances that are not always clear they cause a build up in the gut or induce other problems such as blackhead.

Thread Worms can infect the whole bird.

Mucosa become thickened, the intestines are destroyed and frequently the birds will die. Tapeworms cause slow growth, listlessness in the flock and low egg production. Sometimes they are visible in droppings, but frequently they create a mass which actually blocks the intestines.

Gapeworms are found in the trachea causing grunting (gapes), open mouths and noisy breathing.

Dealing with worms is a twofold process. Firstly, it is best to let the hens have a new piece of land to scratch on every couple of months. The life cycle of these worms includes other animals such as earthworms, slugs, snails and insects; in fact everything hens love to eat. If you can interrupt this life cycle from the hen to the soil and then into another carrier and finally back into the hen, then you will cut down the burden for the hens.

Secondly, you should worm your hens regularly, at least once every six weeks. It is a simple matter to put a measured dose of wormer into the feed. Combined, these two processes should be sufficient to keep worms and internal parasites down to a minimum.

Marek's Disease

Otherwise known as MD, it is likely that infected poultry will die and that the rest of your flock will become infected. MD is a world-wide killer of poultry that has disastrous effects. It is a viral disease similar to herpes.

Symptoms

This disease first appears to be like a cancer in the hen. It is likely that you will notice it in the eyes of the bird, with the iris becoming granular. They then start to fall about because the nervous system is infected, leading to tumors. Then, due to their sick state, they will begin to fall prey to various other diseases.

Birds, once they have the disease, will remain infectious. The virus stays on dust and the main route of infection is actually via dust. Young hatch completely free of the virus, so it is possible to incubate eggs and have clean stock again, but they must not be kept together with infected adult birds.

There is no known treatment for Marek's disease and vaccination is the best method of prevention. Unfortunately the virus mutates very quickly in much the same way as the common cold and flu.

Prevention is almost the only way we can keep this disease at bay. Excellent hygiene is an absolute must and the flow of poultry for commercial reasons needs to be in an all in, all out system. It is likely that people contemplating a broiler unit will not have hens long enough for this disease to develop, but complete disinfecting between batches of poultry is important. New birds = new start.

Mixing young birds with older ones should not take place until they are at least at point of lay so that their immune systems are fully developed. Wherever possible, try not to mingle birds with a weak immune system with older ones. If there is a problem anywhere the youngsters will get sick very quickly.

For the domestic keeper regular cleaning of sheds and not allowing insects to build up near the hens is important. Try not to allow the birds to drink from puddles. More than anything else, be sure of the quality of the birds you buy, especially from poultry units and rescue centres. A good look in the eye will tell you the bird's status – look for a granular iris.

Coccidiosis

These are microscopic parasites that live more or less everywhere, but in soil in particular, and hens take in a lot of soil in their scratching and feeding. When conditions are not good for coccidia they simply enclose themselves in a hard shell and wait until conditions improve. When a hen ingests one of the 7 types of coccidia that like to live inside their digestive system, the chances of the animal becoming sick depend on a number of factors. Frequently a healthy hen can have great immunity against coccidia, but if there are other problems such as worms or a heavy mite load, or the animal is moulting, then coccidia can build up and start to cause problems.

Coccidiosis is characterised by scruffy looking birds that do not move much. They stand in the corner of the hut and simply look miserable. They will have bloody poo and they can easily die in this state. From there they discharge the lining of the intestine to get rid of the coccidia, but by this time the hen will have necrotic enteritis and should be put down.

It must be emphasised that hens with coccidial problems will often fall prey to other diseases because their immune system will be seriously debilitated.

Treatments and Coccidiostats

The most important part of the treatment is prevention by not allowing pasture to build up coccidia. Move your hens frequently, change their bedding frequently and always make sure their drinking water is in perfect condition. If you wouldn't drink it, why should they? Maintain dry conditions and remove puddles and wet bedding. In wet conditions the coccidia will have shed their hard protective cysts and they are much more active in this state.

There are two kinds of drug available. Coccidiostats inhibit the growth of the parasites in the cells of the gut. Coccidiocidals kill the parasites as they make their passage through the gut. If you suspect coccidiosis your vet will have to inspect your birds so that a diagnosis can be made and the appropriate drugs prescribed, which are simply added to the drinking water. You must treat the whole flock. Sick birds may need help to drink, but will respond.

Mycoplasma

This is the result of a single celled organism, now classified as a bacterium, with a very thin cell wall. Generally speaking, the agent invades the respiratory system and the bird looks as though it has a heavy cold. There is frequent sneezing and raspy breathing.

This is not bird flu as the animal would have died within 24 hours. You will, however, need to visit the vet and buy the appropriate antibiotics.

Bird Flu

You may be able to see a certain amount of blueness around the wattles and comb, a condition called cyanosis. You might find hens looking ill, standing still and not eating. They can get a droopy head and look more like vultures than hens. But most likely you will see hens falling dead, and very quickly. If you have numerous unexplained deaths you should contact your vet straight away.

This is a viral disease and must be reported as it is a notifiable disease. It will have dreadful consequences for flocks in your vicinity, but these are necessary steps. Thankfully, this problem is not common in Europe and you are very unlikely to encounter this disease.

Calcium Deficiency

Birds not fed on a balanced ration can suddenly start pulling their feathers out, especially on the belly. They scratch incessantly and are unable to keep still. This problem can also develop with birds fed a balanced ration, but unable to absorb calcium from it.

The treatment is simple. A couple of pots of probiotic yoghurt will have them back to normal within a couple of days, though it will take longer to regrow the feathers.

Aspergillosis

This disease is caused by fungal spores from aspergillum and found mostly in young birds kept on infected litter. There is little that can be done for these birds, which become thirsty and sometimes cough a lot. They seldom last more than a couple of months, but they are not generally infectious in small flocks. In a large flock they may pass on the disease.

Fowl Pox

This is a viral infection that you should not see if you bought your hens from a reputable breeder or you have ex-battery hens. The virus causes lesions on the skin and mouth and sometimes in the airway, which can scab over. This problem can be immunised against when the birds are young, so be sure where you buy from. It is not treatable.

Infectious Bronchitis

Birds look as though they have a great flu. They shiver, don't eat and sneeze and cough. They will all catch the disease as it is highly infectious. The health of the birds before they get ill will dictate how well they get over the problem and they will remain infectious for many weeks after they begin to look better. You will probably lose some birds, but the addition of an antibiotic in the drinking water will help keep down secondary infections.

Newcastle Disease

This viral infection is a notifiable disease that can be immunised against, but, like viruses, genetic changes can mean new strains appear. The birds will all catch the disease within a few days of each other. There is a nasal discharge and often a discharge from the mouth. The eyes go cloudy too as the virus builds up.

Wings can become awkwardly positioned due to paralysis, and the head is often held in an unusual way. They may die or recover, but there is little you can do. Normally birds are vaccinated, so it should never really occur in ordinary flocks.

A Final Thought

There are many preparations on the market that look as though they will keep birds healthy. They often imply that they help to keep internal parasites to a minimum and promote wellbeing. Many are garlic-based and some have essential oils and added vitamins.

It should, however, be noted that, although these preparations will not harm your flock, and indeed may well do what they say, helping to keep birds healthy because they provide nutrients and chemicals that do restrict some parasites, they are not in any way designed to replace correct wormers, coccidiostats, and appropriate veterinary intervention.

Use them by all means, but do not expect them to replace the vet. Nor will they make up for poor quality living conditions and poor food and water that you yourself wouldn't drink.

DIAGNOSTIC GUIDE TO CHICKEN AILMENTS AND TREATMENT		
Signs of Disease	Causes	Treatment & Prevention
HEAD AND NECK		
Crossed beak, top beak overgrown.	Genetic, nutritional.	Might be an inherited defect. Trim to shape. Check diet.
Listless, eyes dull and lifeless.	Part of any general disease.	Check for other symptoms.
Eye discharge, one eye or both.	Local infection as a result of dust or environmental factors/bacterial infection. Part of generalized infection such as Mycoplasmosis. Look for other symptoms.	Bathe the eye with saline solution and treat with antibiotic eye drops or cream. If Mycoplasmosis treat with a soluble antibiotic such as Tylosin.
Eyes sunk into sockets.	Dehydration usually due to diarrhoea. Need to determine the cause of the diarrhoea.	Make sure a plentiful supply of clean drinking water is available until a diagnosis is made.
Comb and wattle pale and looking anaemic.	May just be immaturity if youngster and comb small.	
	External parasites (red mite, lice).	Treat for red mite and lice with pyrethrum powder. Spray house with cypermethrin.
	Internal parasites.	Anthelmintic in the feed usually for up to 7 days.
White scabs and flakey.	Scaly face or Favus. Fungal infection. Microsporum gallinae.	Use gloves and rub in athlete's foot cream for 7 days. Avoid the eyes. Treat premises with Virkon or F10.
Purple comb when normally red.	Heart failure due to age/overweight.	Individual treatment possible. See vet.
	Nitrate poisoning.	Methylene blue in water.
	Severe respiratory distress.	Needs further diagnosis.
Nasal discharge with sneezing.	Dusty environment.	Improve ventilation and get rid of dust.
	Probable general infection such as Mycoplasmosis. Needs further diagnosis.	Soluble antibiotic in the drinking water, depending on the cause.
Swollen sinus(es).	Part of general infection/Mycoplasmosis.	Soluble antibiotic, depending on the cause.
Ears: cheese like substance in ear canal.	Bacterial or mite infection.	Olive oil drops or (not licensed for use), dog ear drops - need to consult vet.
Cheese-like material in mouth and back of throat.	Canker due to Trichomonas infection.	Metronidazole in the water. Vitamin supplement.

Signs of Disease	Causes	Treatment and Prevention
SKIN AND FEATHERS		
Losing feathers.	Normal moult. Usually 3-4 weeks in late summer/early autumn.	Check nutrition. May need supplementation if prolonged.
Feather pecking often with vent pecking.	Feather pecking, bullying. May cause bleeding and death if not stopped. Overcrowding and stress can be factors.	Isolate culprit, usually the bird with all its feathers remaining. Check environment. Treat wounds with coloured antibiotic spray or Stockholm tar.
Losing feathers and itchy.	External parasites: red mite, lice.	Pyrethrum powder over birds and perches. Treat house with cypermethrin. Fipronil dog flea spray (not licensed) can be sprayed on a cloth and wiped on individual birds.
Raised, crusty lesions on legs. 'Scaly leg.'	Skin mites.	Dunk legs in surgical spirit weekly or Avermectin drops on the skin. Not licensed for poultry. See the vet.
Nasty smell with scabby, inflamed vent with yellow discharge.	'Vent Gleet' as a result of Herpes virus infection.	Aciclovir (not licensed for poultry) but probably better to cull as keeps recurring.
Spoiling around the vent or pasted around the vent.	Any form of diarrhoea (see below).	Diagnosis required for treatment.
Pendulous crop.	Crop bound usually due to poor, over fibrous diet. Usually older birds.	Isolate and starve with water only for 48 hours. May require surgery in extreme cases.
Swollen crop with sour smell, bird lethargic.	Sour crop due to yeast infection.	Oral Ketoconizole. Not licensed -needs vet.
BREATHING		
Rapid breathing with eye and nasal discharge and swollen sinuses.	Mycoplasmosis.	Soluble antibiotic such as Tylosin. Use Virkon or equivalent to disinfect premises.
Increased breathing rate, often with reduced egg quality (wrinkled shells).	Infectious bronchitis due to corona virus infection. High mortality possible in the young.	No treatment. Vaccination is effective as prevention. Adults may be carriers.
Breathing distress with gasping and death.	Aspergillosis - fungal infection like 'Farmers Lung.' Affects mostly young poultry. (NB. could infect people).	Cull affected birds, treat environment. Get rid of damp litter. Nebulise with F10 disinfectant.
Large numbers of birds gasping, sick and dying with eye and nasal discharge, comb and wattles often very dark.	Avian (Bird) flu/several viruses, varying pathogenicity. Highly infectious. (NB. notifiable disease and possibly infectious to people).	Blood test required to confirm.

Signs of Disease	Causes	Treatment and Prevention
BREATHING CONTINUED		
Gasping or gaping breathing with diarrhoea.	Gape worms. Syngamus trachea.	Anthelmintic daily in the feed for 7 days - Flubendazole. Eggs must not be consumed for 7 days from the end of treatment. Same for meat.
DIARRHOEA		
Diarrhoea white in colour with perhaps some blood. Young birds over 21 days old.	Coccidiosis, usually Eimeria species.	Coccidiostats eg. Toltrazuril (Baycox), Sulphadimethoxine (Coxi Plus), Amprolium (Coxoid) in water for 5 days. Make sure litter is dry. To prevent put coccidiostat in feed.
White diarrhoea - often fatal in young birds.	Salmonella pullorum. Needs bacteriology and blood tests to diagnose. Salmonella typhinurium/ enteritidis. (NB. notifiable disease with potential to infect people).	Antibiotic - see vet. Cull adult carriers. Clean up environment. Vaccination is possible.
Yellow diarrhoea, mostly turkeys and pheasants. Uncommon in chickens. Can be high mortality in turkeys and pheasants.	Blackhead caused by protozoa. Histomonas parasite carried by intestinal worm Heterakis gallinarum. Mostly affects turkeys, but Heterakis worm is carried by chickens.	Treat with metronidazole in water for 5 days. Worm hens to get rid of intermediate host, Heterakis. Never keep chickens and turkeys together.
Green colour diarrhoea.	Too much green food, especially cabbage.	Check diet.
Green colour diarrhoea and listless - all poultry.	Intestinal parasitic worms.	Flubendazole in feed for 7 days. Should treat twice a year. Eggs and meat cannot be consumed for 7 days after treatment. Clean environment.
Green diarrhoea along with respiratory and nervous symptoms.	Newcastle disease/Fowl pest due to paramyxovirus infection (NB. notifiable disease).	Uk is mostly clear of disease. Recommend only to vaccinate in face of outbreak.
Brown diarrhoea in young birds from about 5 days old.	E. coli infection. Stress factors/cold and dirty wet litter.	Soluble antibiotic in water for up to a week. Oxytetracycline and apramycin. Improve environment.
LAMENESS		
Swelling on foot, mostly underside.	Bumblefoot, usually bacterial infection in older, heavy birds.	Antibiotic and poulticing. May need surgery. Guarded outlook for recovery.
Paralysis, same side wing and leg.	Mareks disease due to a Herpes virus. Various strains.	Cull affected birds. No effective treatment. Vaccinate. Keep youngsters away from possible adult carriers.

Signs of Disease	Causes	Treatment and Prevention
LAMENESS CONTINUED		
Non-specific lameness.	Injury or tumour or arthritis. Kidney disease.	Needs more diagnosis before treatment. If injury and not fracture then complete rest will be indicated.
	Potential fracture.	Would need vet input. Many simple fractures can be splinted.
	Perosis due to bird growing too rapidly to allow sufficient calcium and phosphorus in the bones.	Check nutrition/reduce protein in diet. Check vitamin and mineral content of the diet.
	Lameness in one or both legs may be due to internal parasites.	Check faeces for parasite eggs and treat with Flubendazole in feed for 7 days, if positive.
Swollen hocks.	Arthritis or Mycoplasma infection.	Antibiotic such as Tylosin or Lincomycin if infection diagnosed. For non-infective causes use non-steroidal anti-inflammatory drugs eg. Meloxican. NB. not licensed and need to see vet.
	In young birds deformation of bones and joints may indicate metabolic disease due to calcium/phosphorus imbalance in diet.	Check diet with vet/nutritionalist and rectify if necessary.
Splay legs.	Common problem in newly hatched. Could be nutritional or slippery surface.	Tie legs together with soft wool for 2-3 days, but not usually successful and would need to cull.
Deformities.	Common inheritied deformities. Roach back (Kyphosis), Scoliosis, cow hocks, inwardly bent toes.	Most birds with severe deformities should be culled.
BEHAVIOUR		
Weight loss but still bright and feeding.	Nutritional ie. inadequate diet.	Check diet.
	Intestinal worms.	Flubendazole daily in food for 7 days. Eggs and meat must not be consumed for 7 days from the end of treatment.
	Avian Tuberculosis (NB. potential to infect people).	No treatment. Cull affected birds.
Any change in flock or individual behaviour.	May be stress related.	Dim lights if possible. Shut in shed for a time if possible. Apply vitamins and probiotics.

Signs of Disease	Causes	Treatment and Prevention
ADULT SUDDEN DEATH		
Without prior warning.	Need post-mortem. Consider predator eg. fox, mink etc. Egg Peritonitis. Result of yolk in abdomen missing oviduct. Heart failure. Kidney failure. Aspergillosis. Botulism. Newcastle disease (NB. notifiable disease).	Probable most common cause of sudden death.
	Poisoning: blue green algae. Plant poisoning or chemical poisons eg. arsenic, lead, slug bait, pesticides.	Keep water containers clean, stop access to stagnant water. Check for and remove: laburnum seeds, potato sprouts, black nightshade, henbane, iris, privet, rhododendron, oleander, yew, caster oil, sweet pea, rapeseed, clematis, St. John's wort, vetch, ragwort, rhubarb leaves and some fungi.
YOUNG SUDDEN DEATH		
Without prior warning.	Consider predator eg. fox. Smothering.	Poor environment - too hot or cold or panic causing excessive crowding together.
	Gumboro Disease (infectious Bursitis).	Vaccinate breeding birds, can protect chicks.
	Salmonellosis. Newcastle Disease.	
EGG LAYING		
Laying adult birds - no eggs.	Fright or stress - new home. Laying away. Rats or birds stealing eggs. Infectious Bronchitis. Egg eating by hens.	Scatter table tennis balls or golf balls or china eggs as a deterrent or make nest boxes darker.
No eggs, listless and straining in individual adults.	Egg bound. Remove if possible but this can lead to prolapse.	Need vet if prolapsed - emergency procedure. Calcium and oxytocin injection may be required. Cull if bird has egg peritonitis.
Prolapsed vent/oviduct.	Usually found dead due to pecking by companions. Age, stress and overweight can be precipitating factors.	No cure possible. Surgery not practical if found alive.

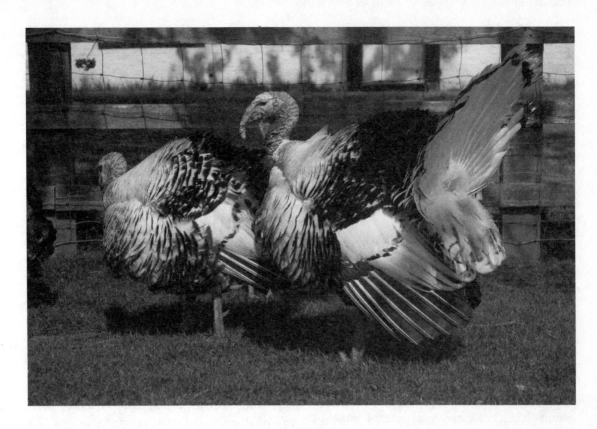

Chapter Three

TURKEYS - INJURIES, AILMENTS AND PARASITES

By Janice Houghton-Wallace

You could be forgiven for reading a chapter with this title and thinking that keeping turkeys is really difficult and perhaps not for you. Yes, some of the diseases are unpleasant and some could result in fatalities. Very few turkeys will, however, experience the problems described here and, if they are looked after in a correct manner, they will most certainly live a long and healthy life without being afflicted by any of them.

However, every responsible turkey keeper should be aware of how their birds can become sick, because turkeys can suffer un-

necessarily if the owner does not realise there is a problem. The sooner any illness or injury is recognised, the sooner that any possible treatment can be given and the better chance the bird will have of making a full recovery. Once a bird is ailing it does need to be dealt with immediately, as it takes time for any veterinary treatment to begin working and during that time the bird is still losing condition. Therefore one of the best pieces of advice that can be given is to get to know your turkeys. This may seem a rather strange remark, but let me put it another way. Time spent just looking at and being with your birds is never time wasted. You will begin to recognise how they look and behave when they are in the best of health. You will get used to seeing them forage or play in a particular way and will become aware of how much and how often they eat and drink or communicate. Then, when a turkey doesn't react in the way that you are used to seeing, it is usually a sign that something isn't quite right and should be investigated further. This is simply applying good stockmanship and is a valuable skill to develop.

To remain fit all birds need to have shelter from inclement weather, nutritious feed, fresh water and a clean, stimulating environment. If you can provide these then you will have gone a long way to contributing towards maintaining your turkeys' health. However, just like humans, they do occasionally have things the matter with them that you perhaps had not expected. These can be injuries, a malaise brought on through a change of location, activity, even tiredness, or a bacterial, parasitic or viral infection. Ill health may well be infectious, but equally it could be nutritional, a gut or reproductive system disturbance or a dysfunction as in crop impaction, or a prolapse.

Aspergillosis

This is a fungal disease caused by Aspergillus fumigatus. It affects mainly young poults and typical symptoms are gasping for breath, weakness, thirst and drowsiness. The infection causes eye lesions in older birds. A respiratory disease, it is caught through inhaling spores from damp or mouldy litter or feed. Good hygiene is essential to eliminate this problem. Always replace damp litter with dry, dust free quality litter, clean feeders regularly and do not allow stale feed to accumulate in the corners of feeders or feed to spill onto litter which then goes mouldy over time. There is no real cure for this disease. Nystatin, a human medicine that can be accessed via a veterinary

surgeon may be worth considering, but is not always effective.

Avian Influenza (fowl plague)

Avian influenza, commonly called bird flu, is a notifiable contagious disease affecting the respiratory, digestive and/or nervous system of any species of bird and causes exceptionally high mortality, especially in turkeys. The cause is a virus, Orthomyxovirus type A, and highly pathogenic forms (HPAI) are usually of the H groups 5 and 7. The symptoms of HPAI are quite dramatic, with one of the very first signs being a sudden high death rate. Other signs include a loss of appetite, a drop in egg production, a nasal and ocular discharge, a swollen face, the combs and wattle turning dark blue-black, depression, coughing and paralysis. The low pathogenic (LPAI) form of the disease commonly causes only mild symptoms such as ruffled feathers, a drop in egg production and some respiratory signs, but the disease could go completely undetected. Transmission is through direct contact with secretions from infected birds, especially faeces, contaminated feed, water, equipment and clothing. Poults may themselves be affected by broken contaminated eggs in the incubator.

A veterinary surgeon should be called in if there is any suspicion of avian influenza. Do not take the bird to the veterinary practice in case it is avian influenza as the risk of spreading the disease must be considered. The vet or the owner must then directly notify the Department for Environment, Food and Rural Affairs (Defra) if it looks as though it could be avian influenza and the Animal Health will be called in to assess the situation and take tests for laboratory analysis.

There is no treatment or preventive at present in the UK as vaccination can only be done with European Commission approval through

Defra. Any infected birds in an outbreak are culled. To reduce the risk of avian influenza turkey keepers are advised to keep feed under cover to minimise the attraction to wild birds, keep water fresh and free of droppings, keep waterfowl away from turkeys, control vermin, isolate new stock for two to three weeks, isolate turkeys for fourteen days if they have been taken to an exhibition, change clothes and wash boots before and after visiting other breeders and their flocks or before and after attending a poultry sale, keep fresh disinfectant at the entrance to poultry areas for dipping footwear or have plastic overboots available, disinfect crates before and after use, disinfect vehicles which have been on poultry premises (avoid taking vehicles onto other premises if possible), wash hands before and after handling your turkeys and comply with any import/export regulations/guidelines.

Avian Tuberculosis

Avian tuberculosis is a bacterial infection caused by Mycobacterium avium and, although rare, is seen in turkeys kept outdoors which have close contact with wild birds. Transmission is through infected faeces, contamination and fomites (inanimate objects capable of transmitting infection eg. clothing). The infected bird will lose a great deal of weight, eventually becoming emaciated. It may also become lame and have diarrhoea. Although this is a very serious disease with no effective treatment, it is possible for a single bird only to be affected in a small group. Confirmation of avian tuberculosis is at post-mortem. A veterinary surgeon might do a post-mortem on a turkey carcass for you which would show yellow nodules on the intestine and other internal organs, even bone marrow if the bird died of avian tuberculosis. The regional Veterinary Laboratories Agency may also carry out post-mortems on fresh avian carcasses. There would be a fee for any post-mortems undertaken.

Blackhead (see Worms)

Breast Blisters

Blisters on the keel bone are caused by inflammation and infection with Staphylococcus bacteria. This can be brought on through leg problems and turkeys continually sitting down on wet or soiled litter. Any leg problems should always be addressed, but clean, dry litter is equally important. Breast blisters can also be a symptom of Mycoplasma synoviae infection.

Broken Bones

Turkey bones are quite brittle, so landing on hard surfaces from a height without room to glide down gently is never satisfactory. If a turkey breaks a bone it may be possible to mend it under a surgical procedure, but this can be expensive and there are very few veterinary surgeons able or willing to carry out such operations on this species. The recuperation process will take many weeks of very careful nursing.

I once had a Bourbon Red stag called Biscuit. He had broken his femur but was operated on at the Queen's Veterinary School Hospital at the University of Cambridge and made a full recovery. Orthopaedic Surgeon Sorrel Langley-Hobbs joined the broken bone with a three inch pin and four screws in an operation that took nearly three hours to complete. It was a first for Sorrel and her team, but she believed it was worth a try and it proved to be the right decision because the operation was successful and much was learnt about avian bone surgery. As this procedure had not been carried out before on a turkey, Sorrel wrote a paper about the operation which was published in

The Veterinary Record, the British Veterinary Association's journal.

The fact that Biscuit was used to being handled and his resulting placid temperament certainly contributed to the successful outcome. Had he not been used to close human contact then the operation may not have taken place at all because it would have been far too stressful. Of course, such extreme veterinary attention is not an everyday solution, but it is quite amazing what can be done for a particular pet.

Broken Claws

A broken claw can occur during perching at any age if the bird catches itself awkwardly when turning or descending. This can produce quite a lot of blood and can be quite frightening if red splashes are seen on perches, walls, litter etc., before you have established what the cause is. Never ignore an open wound, however small, because, even though the environment may appear relatively clean, there will be bacteria lurking everywhere and the last thing you want is an infection getting into the wound. With no prevention this can happen in a matter of days with the toe and foot swelling and becoming increasingly painful. The bird then begins to limp because it feels uncomfortable and this then puts it at risk of being bullied by other members of the flock. As soon as you find a bird with a broken claw which has completely detached itself, spray the area with an antibiotic. Terramycin is good for this purpose as it gets into every crevice. Should the claw still be partly hanging, clip it off if it can be done without injuring the bird further, and treat it. If the toe has already begun to swell or is only partly severed, then a visit to the vet is the best option. If such a wound is left unattended infection can do a great deal of damage and a veterinary surgeon may have no choice but to amputate the toe.

Bumblefoot

Bumblefoot is a problem which can occur through descending from too high a perch onto a hard surface, causing bruising of the pad, or through a chronic wound that fails to heal. As the injury worsens the lesion enlarges until the foot is greatly distended, particularly the underneath, which is usually ulcerated. This swelling is caused by Staphylococci bacteria entering the lesion. It is difficult to treat but antibiotic use will help prevent any further infection developing in the bird and may ease the condition. In extreme cases the ulcerated part breaks away and it is possible to remove a thickened core from the pad. This should immediately be cleansed with antibiotic spray to prevent any further infection from entering. Recovery from bumblefoot takes a long time but, if the suspected cause of the injury is removed and the bird is kept on soft, clean litter, it may well overcome the problem.

Cannibalism

This is a behavioural problem that can cause slight injury, severe injury or even death, depending on how soon it is noticed. There are different forms manifested through different reasons. At the youngest stage in life it can be seen through self-inflicting wounds in poults, when they peck at their feet. This is unusual but can happen in one poult in a group. Whatever has triggered the predicament, the poult obviously feels an irritation and pecks at the problem, eventually making the area raw and producing blood, which exacerbates the situation, especially when other poults join in. As it is extremely unusual for the complete group to be affected it is difficult to ascertain the cause. Normally it would be overcrowding, excessive light, too high a temperature, poor feed quality or simply boredom. Check that bedding is clean, ventilation good and the environment not too hot. Although they cannot be prescribed as treatments because neither are licensed for use on poultry, I have found that for a poult that is pecking a toe, rubbing some Germolene or Conotrane on the wound helps to anaesthetise the area and heal the wound. After a few days of treatment the condition has disappeared. This problem may lead on from feather pecking (see separate heading).

The worst form of cannibalism is when turkeys set upon one of their group and 'mug' it endlessly, to death if allowed. The pecking usually takes place around the head and neck area until this part of the body is completely raw, covered in blood and damaged skin tissue. The victim should be removed immediately if this type of serious bullying is suspected. If noticed soon enough the bird can be treated with antibiotic powder and isolated and recovery can be complete after about a fortnight. If left too long the bird is best put out of its misery, or in extreme cases may actually die of its injuries. The best thing to do if this occurs is to change the environment of the other birds. A change of house or transferring to accommodation where they can get outside on grass, with a more interesting environment, can solve the problem. If this cannot be done, try to enrich the environment in the house by hanging up some vegetation for them to peck. Sometimes it helps to hang up objects that shine or move, such as CDs, which will give them something to investigate. Do make sure that any string hung up does not have lose ends and is high enough for them not to try to eat it and choke!

If there is one particular bully in the group it may well be worth considering isolating it or despatching it. However, the problem with removing birds from a group is that occasionally the 'second in command' sees the main bully gone and simply takes its place, reinforcing the behaviour. Also, it is an extraordinary fact that a turkey being bullied, if put in a different environment, is quite capable of turning round and bullying the others. If isolated but with neighbours through a fence, it will try to fight with the bird on the other side, especially a male in springtime. It is possible to reintroduce a bird without any adverse effects, but do be prepared for some sparring.

Coccidiosis

Coccidiosis is caused by a small gut parasite, Eimeria , which can affect poults from two to sixteen weeks of age, but is more often seen in those at three to six weeks. There are seven species of Eimeria which infect turkeys, but only two tend to cause disease; Eimeria meleagrimitis which affects the upper small intestine and Eimeria adenoides affecting the caecae and rectum. Symptoms are drooping wings, ruffled feathers, listless, depressed appearance and watery diarrhoea which can be blood stained or have lumps of blood or mucus in it. Toltrazuril, Sulphonamides or Amprolium are veterinary treatments that can be used. As yet there is no specific Coccidiosis vaccine for turkeys in the UK and the chicken vaccine doesn't work on turkeys. Good hygiene is immensely important. The housing, especially the flooring, should be cleansed and disinfected thoroughly before poults are placed there. Any damp litter, particularly around drinkers, should be replaced immediately with dry, clean litter. Biosecurity is also important because of the possibility of transferring Coccidia oocysts from infected faeces via footwear. A coccidiostat (preventive medicine) may be available in proprietary feed but do beware; do not be tempted to feed medicated chicken feed to turkeys as some chicken medications are toxic for turkeys.

Crop Impaction

This can happen through the eating of very long grass which doesn't pass through the crop properly and begins to bind up the contents. Although there are solutions which can be tried at home it is better to consult a veterinary surgeon who may have to surgically remove the mass. Birds do recover but the possibility of it happening again should be remembered and consideration given to where the bird is allowed to graze. The condition can also suggest a blockage further down the intestine leading to stasis, eg. gizzard impaction or MOGPID (Mass of Grass Protruding Into the Duodenum). This is more likely to occur in spring when there is long, lush grass which impacts and could also lead to fermentation in the crop. Because of the risk of fermentation grass cuttings should never be given to turkeys. In a separate condition the crop can become pendulous, whereby it hangs below the normal breast line. Although the cause may be similar to crop impaction, here the muscles are so weak that they are unable to process the food. If this arises consult a vet.

Curled Toe

Occasionally a poult can have a curled toe at hatching. This can be as a result of a genetic defect or a temperature fluctuation during artificial incubation. The condition can also suggest a mineral or vitamin deficiency in the mother failing to pass on sufficient into the egg. Although very fiddly this can be addressed with a tiny splint made of a slither of matchstick and some tape. Medical tape which allows the skin to breathe is better than other kinds, but you only need a very small piece and ideally it should be replaced every two or three days to allow for growth. This minute splint will help to straighten the toe during its early development and, after a fortnight or

so, can be removed by which time the toe has usually corrected itself. Any such splints must be light and constantly checked for chafing.

Egg Peritonitis

During the laying season a turkey could possibly suffer from egg peritonitis. This is when something goes wrong with the egg tube or the egg inside the bird, which consequently cannot be laid. The yolk may miss the funnel of the infundibulum, or the shell may be misshapen and become stuck. The egg may break, introducing infection into the body or it will simply sit in the cavity, eventually becoming toxic. In either case peritonitis will kill the bird. It is possible to diagnose this problem, especially if the hen turkey is in a laying cycle but has suddenly stopped. She will be showing signs of great discomfort and possibly opening and closing her beak as though panting very slowly. This is a symptom of being in great pain. If you handle the bird very gently without putting any pressure on her sides and feel her underneath, this may be distended and extremely hard, just like the top of a drum. At this stage infection is rife and the turkey should be put out of her misery as there is nothing that can be done for peritonitis. This ailment is more common in spring when birds come into sexual activity at the start of the laying season.

Egg Bound

This is when a turkey cannot pass the egg comfortably and is similar to constipation. She will stand hunched up and possibly straining at the same time. This is a type of cramp and can be a result of a lack of calcium in the diet or stress. The turkey should be isolated in a warm place and, if possible, put a little warm olive oil in the vent. If the egg is partially showing then a veterinary surgeon should be consulted.

Erysipelas

Erysipelothrix insidiosa can occasionally be seen in poults and adult turkeys. Among the signs are sudden death, or the bird may have a swollen snood, a chronic scabby skin, lameness and depression. Poults have swollen joints. The bacterium can enter through scratches in the skin where stags have been fighting and hence it is seen in stags more than in hens. It can live in the soil for many years and there is an increased risk of it occurring in turkeys if they are kept on land previously used for pigs or sheep. The condition can be treated with antibiotics and good hygiene should keep it at bay. One of the essential aspects of a clean environment is good vermin control. Rats and mice can induce and spread disease, so an eradication programme should be put in place to dispose of them.

Favus

These are small whitish growths found on the head and neck caused by the fungus Trichophyton gallinae. The problem is quite rare and usually associated with unhygienic conditions such as stale, dirty litter and unclean feeders and drinkers. It can be treated by mixing formalin in petroleum jelly and, using a rubber glove, gently rubbing it onto the skin.

Feather Pecking

Feather pecking is a vice usually seen in birds confined in too small an area or in an environment that offers too little stimulation. Turkeys do like to have interest in their day and if boredom overcomes them they will make their own interest, and what they come up with may not be very pleasant. Feather pecking around the neck and vent area is most common. This can begin through birds cleaning their beaks on another turkey's feathers or through boredom, but often the birds will eat the feathers, suggesting that their diet may have something to do with it, for feathers are a form of protein. This behavioural pattern can range from just a few feathers going missing around the neck or tail to complete feathers being destroyed and severe injury on the back of a bird, with the base of the back becoming devoid of any feathers and blood being drawn. Enrich the birds' environment, because if not addressed this could lead to cannibalism. Check over the birds for mites because it could be that irritation is causing them to peck at the feathers themselves, which then encourages others to do the same. Provide a good dust-bathing area, although you will notice that if internal accommodation is cleaned regularly turkeys just love dust-bathing in fresh shavings. In the summer they will find a good dry piece of soil outside and this will become their dust bath.

Fighting

As winter turns to spring males can become quite feisty with one another. This is perfectly normal and it is the natural process for determining which genes will be carried forward into the next generation. Even if a group of males have grown up together and have no females around, they will still go through the basic seasonal routine of 'hormones out of control,' which usually involves being beastly to their best friends! Stag fights can cause injury but for most of the time these pass without too much of a problem. They will scar each other on the head and eventually one will take a back seat, allowing the other to be 'master.' Any serious fighting and damage should immediately be dealt with and the victim removed.

If the scratches are really bad it can allow bacteria to enter wounds, so treatment with an antibiotic powder or spray is certainly wise. Full thickness skin tears can lead to large gaping wounds which may need veterinary attention and stitching together. Occasionally, hen turkeys will also fight and this can be quite dramatic for a few days but again, just keep an eye on the situation and they will usually settle down after a while and become the best of pals again. Once separated, especially for more than one to two days, be prepared for fights and bullying on reintroduction. This is why care has to be taken when reintroducing a bird and the best time to attempt this is at dusk when they can then sleep together under the same roof before venturing out together in daylight. If trying to introduce birds that haven't previously lived together it is worth putting them all into a new environment so that they all have something unaccustomed to get used to.

Fowl Cholera

Fowl cholera is a highly infectious disease caused by the bacterium Pasteurella multocida. It can range from acute septicaemia to chronic and localised infections, along with swollen joints, lameness, coughing and ruffled feathers, but is usually first noticed by sudden death. The infection can be present in rodents, so it is essential that effective pest control is undertaken. Sulphonamides, tetracyclines, erythromycin, streptomycin and penicillin can be used in treatment, but the disease can reoccur so treatment can take a long time to be effective.

Haemorrhagic Enteritis

This is a viral disease which results in heavy bleeding in the intestine. The turkeys go off their feed and water and have diarrhoea. Bleeding can be seen from the vent just prior to death. Causes of the disease can be unsuitable feed, contaminated water, a sudden change of environment or poor husbandry.

Turkeys can become affected if outside in inclement weather with little or no protection. Treat it with oral tetracycline and the bird will need isolating in a warm, clean and peaceful environment for up to four weeks. There is no effective 'treatment' as this is a viral disease but TLC may facilitate recovery. It is often first recognised as a result of sudden death, but closed groups can often build up an immunity to this disease, so it may just affect a recently introduced stressed bird.

Hexamitiasis

Hexamita meleagridis is a protozoan parasite transmitted by faeces, fomites and carriers. The bird loses its appetite, then weight and passes a watery diarrhoea before becoming very depressed, eventually going into a coma. Convulsions may take place before death. Tetracycline is used to treat this disease and the bird should be kept in a warm, comfortable environment. If antibiotics are given this is to control any secondary bacteria that may be present. Good hygiene helps to reduce the risk of hexamitiasis, especially regular changing of drinking water and thorough scrubbing of drinkers or troughs. It may result from birds drinking from dirty puddles, so avoid poached areas in pens. The disease can also evolve when groups of turkeys of different ages are mixed.

Leg Problems

Turkeys suffer from various conditions which affect their legs. Perosis is one such condition that can easily be avoided with good nutrition. It is a thickening, shortening and distortion of the bones associated with a deficiency of calcium, phosphorus, manganese and choline in the ration. If turkey poults and growers are given an appropriate proprietary ration for their age this disease should not occur.

Perosis should not be confused with a condition of newly hatched poults called 'spraddle legs.' This is likely to be linked to a fault during incubation or improper diet of the parent stock. In turkeys the metatarsus often turns at a right angle, so the legs are actually splayed. There is no actual cure for this problem but it may be possible to make a small support in the form of a tiny figure of eight tie which draws the hocks together and can, over the course of a week or two, remedy the problem. Then, with correct nutrition, the poult can recover. Any support will need to be changed after a few days to allow for growth and to prevent any restriction.

Adult turkeys could also suffer from a slipped tendon. It is vitally important not to catch turkeys by a single leg because joints can so easily slip out. The worst scenario is that the lameness is caused by a tumour, but the condition of the rest of the bird could well give a clue as to whether this is the problem or not.

There are a number of infections occurring in turkeys that affect legs, so it is not always easy to immediately determine the problem unless other factors are taken into account, or dismissed accordingly. Mycoplasmas can swell the leg joints causing lameness, Ornithobacterium infection (ORT), which has similar symptoms to mycoplasma, can affect the use of the legs, or turkeys can simply sprain or just bruise themselves, which can cause lameness for a while. If, after inspection, disease can be ruled out, then the pain of a sprain or bruising can be eased for a while by giving the turkey a basic aspirin tablet.

Very heavy mature turkeys can develop leg problems. If hybridised turkeys in particular are kept as pets this should be taken into consideration and a suitable diet and plenty of exercise given. Occasionally it is just not possible to work out why a turkey is lame, and even on veterinary inspection no clear diagnosis can be made. Usually a course of antibiotics will be advised and often, with good care, the birds do recover.

Lice

Lice are insects with flattened bodies that live on the skin or feathers of turkeys. They are more often found around the vent area because this is where they find moisture and lay their eggs. Although poults may become susceptible to lice once outside on grass, it is the adult birds and in particular the stags that more readily catch these parasites. Lice are yellowish-brown in colour and can easily be noticed if feathers are parted, especially around the vent, thighs or wings. There are two species of lice that are found specifically on turkeys and three other species that are chicken lice, but if turkeys are kept close to or with the chickens they may catch these as well.

Goniodes Meleagridis (Large turkey louse)

The large turkey louse will be the most commonly found and easiest to spot.

Lipeurus Gallipavonis (Slender turkey louse)

This louse affects turkeys in the same manner as the large turkey louse but this, as with the Liperus heterographus (Chicken head louse), will be seen on close inspection on any part of the turkey, even running around the head of the bird. Eomenacanthus stramineus (Chicken body louse) and Menopon gallianae (Chicken shaft louse) can also transfer to turkeys.

Fortunately all forms of lice can be controlled quite easily with louse powder, but if left untreated they can cause problems. The affected turkeys will gradually lose condition as their health is being challenged and if a stag is heavily infested, especially around the vent area, it may interfere with his ability to mate. If a spot-on parasitical treatment is used it will kill all lice and mites.

Mites

Mites are minuscule eight-legged parasitic insects which can cause great harm and even death if left untreated. Unlike lice, which do not appear to irritate birds greatly, mites will cause considerable irritation, eventually becoming a major welfare problem. Most mites use blood or lymph for food, so anaemia is a constant symptom. Apart from the direct detrimental effect on its host, blood-sucking mites could easily transmit bacterial and viral infections.

Cytodites Nudus (Air-sac mite)

This is a mite that lives as an internal parasite in the bronchi, lungs, air-sacs and bone cavities of birds. It does affect turkeys, but is not really common. The mites are extremely small white specks and how birds become infected is not known. Heavy invasions have been associated with a rapid loss of weight, whereby the birds look very similar to those affected by avian tuberculosis. As the parasite is internal it is difficult to give an accurate diagnosis without a post-mortem and is difficult to treat. A prevention routine such as that for red mite would be useful.

Ermanyssus Gallinae (Red mite)

This troublesome mite is more associated with chickens than turkeys, but turkeys can be affected if kept together with chickens in infected houses. During the daytime these mites live in crevices within the housing and on perches and then climb onto the birds at night, sucking their blood. The red mite can inflict great damage because the birds can become anaemic and will subsequently lose vitality and condition. Always check perches to make sure that no spots of grey powder are present as these are red mite eggs. If these are identified, cleanse the housing thoroughly with products specifically designed to deal with red mite.

Knemidocoptes Mutans (Scaly-leg mite)

The scaly-leg mite lives in the skin of the bird, burrowing underneath the scales on the legs and feet and causing them to lift and form crusts. Turkeys are not as susceptible to this mite as are fowl, but when it does occur the irritation caused is so intense that the birds begin to continually look under their body at their legs, eventually stamping around and pecking at both legs and feet. Petroleum jelly rubbed well into the affected area will help to suffocate the mites. Benzyl benzoate is a white liquid available from veterinary surgeons that can be wiped into the scales in the same way. Eprinex or Ivomec can be used and both are effective, but these treatments are not licensed for poultry. They can be ordered through a vet or a qualified agricultural merchant. It is recommended that you administer no more than seven drops on the skin at the base of the neck for an adult turkey. This treatment will kill all external and many internal parasites. The scales will moult and new ones will grow, which will not be distorted if the mites have been killed. Do not attempt to pull off crusty scales as there will be raw flesh underneath and this will be extremely painful for the bird, with no advantage gained.

Knemidocoptes Gallinae (Depluming mite)

This mite is very similar to the scaly-leg mite and only occasionally infests turkeys. It burrows into the skin beneath the base of the feathers. Treat an infestation with Eprinex drops as for scaly-leg.

Liponyssys Sylviarum (Feather mite)

This can be found living amongst the feathers on the neck and rear of the bird. Anti-mite sprays containing pyrethrum will quickly help the situation, but they can also be treated in the same way as depluming mite.

Moniliasis (see Thrush)

Mycoplasma Gallisepticum (M.G.)

Mycoplasma gallisepticum is a chronic respiratory disease often accompanied by severe sinusitis. It can be passed on through the egg or by direct contact with infected birds and fomites. Turkeys which recover from this disease can remain infected for life, albeit in a dormant form. If the bird then experiences stress or is inflicted in any other way, mycoplasma can recur. A turkey with mycoplasma looks as though it has a very bad cold, with coughing, nasal and eye discharge, swollen sinuses, possible leg problems and a loss of appetite. Antibiotic treatment will be needed but it may help the bird to very gently massage the side of the face toward the beak. Pus will then exude from the nasal opening. Until treatment begins to work the sinus will fill up again, but in the meantime you will have removed at least some of the pressure from the turkey's face, which should make it feel a little more comfortable.

Mycoplasma Iowae (M.I.)

This is a disease which affects unhatched turkey embryos and leads to poor hatchability, the infected embryos being stunted with likely down or feather abnormalities. Infection has largely been removed from commercial breeding stock in the UK.

Mycoplasma Meleagridis (M.M.)

This is a disease causing respiratory and skeletal problems in turkeys. It also causes poor growth in growing birds and reduced hatchability in breeders, leg problems, crooked necks, stunting and slow growth. Transmission is venereal with infection passing through the eggs and it can be brought on through stress and other respiratory infections.

Mycoplasma Synoviae (M.S.)

This is a mild respiratory infection which can become more severe if combined with some other infection. It can lead to coughing, air sac damage, a loss of condition, leg problems and breast blisters. There are different strains of M.S. causing varying degrees of the disease. A blood test is the only way you can be sure that the bird has mycoplasma synoviae.

Good biosecurity is essential to keep any of the mycoplasma infections out of your flock. Always isolate newly bought birds for a fortnight before mixing them. Treatment will reduce the clinical signs, but may not rid the bird of the actual infection. Mycoplasmas are so varied in their susceptibility that the birds may respond more favourably to one antibiotic over another. Tylan, Baytril, Pulmotil AC, Tiamutin, Lincospectin and Aureomycin can each be used. Some are given in the drinking water, others will be injected through the breast muscle.

Mycosis

Mycosis is a term for any disease caused by parasitic fungi. If a piece of skin is affected by fungi it is described as being mycotic. Fungi can attack the unfeathered parts of the head of a turkey. This is called Favus. A yeast-like fungus growing in the lining of the crop or the mouth is called Thrush (Moniliasis) and a fungal infection in the respiratory tract is called Aspergillosis. See under the separate headings.

Newcastle Disease (Fowl pest)

Newcastle Disease is a notifiable disease caused by the virus Paramyxovirus PMV-1. It is highly contagious and the birds exhibit nervous signs and paralysis with loss of appetite, coughing, diarrhoea, depression and a drop in egg production. These symptoms can be associated with other diseases, but the difference here is that the birds will suddenly die and the death of a group of birds should always ring alarm bells. A veterinary surgeon can give a general diagnosis, but laboratory tests will confirm whether or not the birds have contracted Newcastle Disease. This is potentially a very serious viral infection which means that any suspicions must be reported to Defra without delay. In the event of an outbreak, all infected birds are culled and movement restrictions are put in force by Defra. It is possible to vaccinate against Newcastle Disease but it is best to consult your veterinary surgeon as to whether the disease risk in your area is sufficient to warrant this.

PEMS

Poult Enteritis and Mortality Syndrome (PEMS) is an infectious and transmissible viral disease capable of causing sudden or lingering death in poults between seven and twenty eight days of age. It causes gut ache, feed refusal with birds flicking feed out of the feeders and can lead to severe stunting and poor growth. Affected poults show hyperactivity and are more vocal than usual. They drink lots but eat little, becoming increasingly weak. The dropping are a watery pale brown and the birds huddle up together trying to keep warm. A range of antibiotics are useful, but flouroquinolone antimicrobials can also be effective. A good quality poult diet is essential and multivitamins and milk replacers add to the nutritional support. Good hygiene and biosecurity are so important in helping to keep diseases such as PEMS at bay.

Poult Injuries

Growing poults can be quite mischievous and like to jump and fly onto any object they can. Damage can be done during this exploratory phase and it has been known for them to break their necks whilst descending from a height – even a straw bale. It is therefore important not to have anything which can encourage this type of behaviour before they are more fully developed. The natural instinct of getting high to perch overnight is certainly inbuilt and even poults just a fortnight old sometimes try to perch. During the first three months of life a turkey's bones are relatively soft and still developing, so it is best not to allow them to perch, especially on narrow poles, until after this time. This will prevent any denting in the breast bone which could, in later life, make a table bird look less presentable and disqualify an exhibition bird. Bales of straw to jump on are, however, quite acceptable once the poults are at least six or seven weeks old.

Ripped Back

Sometimes hen turkeys are injured during mating. This can be quite traumatic and the injuries may need veterinary attention. Stitches may be required and antibiotics given to stem any infection if the rips are deep. Otherwise scratches can be dealt with by antiseptic powder or spray. Isolate the injured hen from other birds. Turkey breeding saddles should be used on hens that are mating naturally to prevent the male damaging the female whilst he is 'treading' her. A saddle is a 'breakfast plate' sized piece of strong canvas or leather with a semi-circle of thicker strips on the upper part. The stag balances on the saddle and the strips are designed to catch his claws when he treads so that they do not scrape down the sides of the hen.

The saddle sits on the back of the hen and her wings pass through straps that hold the saddle in position. When first in place she may well move around awkwardly for a few minutes trying to unsettle this strange object, but will very soon get used to it and eventually take no notice. A saddle will not restrict the turkey at all. She will still be able to fly, jump, have dust baths and carry out other day to day turkey duties. It is essential to check regularly that her feathers are not covering up any mating damage. Even with a saddle a male can still damage the female if she is knocked sideways and he treads her body, beyond the protection of the saddle.

Salmonella Infections

The term salmonella represents a huge group of bacteria which can infect a large number of animal species including humans. Fortunately only a few are likely to infect poultry and even fewer are associated with disease in turkeys. In most cases the salmonella just sits in the birds' intestines and causes no problems. However, certain types have the capacity to cause disease, especially if your bird is already ailing for some other reason. Salmonella is likely only to really be a problem for young poults.

Although antibiotics may help once a turkey is infected, the approach must always be to reduce the likelihood of infection in the first place. This can be achieved by following the highest standards of hygiene with your birds, but especially by controlling any contact with rats, mice or wild birds. Incidents of salmonella infection associated with certain more significant types have dramatically decreased in recent years following vaccination of commercial flocks.

Salmonella Pullorum (Bacillary white diarrhoea BWD)

Although turkeys of all ages can be affected by salmonella pullorum, it is the very young poults that it can rapidly kill. It is transmitted from affected breeders through the egg. However, it can pass horizontally in young birds and is sometimes associated with cannibalism. The turkeys suffer from a white diarrhoea, depression, ruffled feathers and closed eyes. They cheep loudly, gasp for air and are sometimes lame. Amoxycillin, tetracyclines and flouroquinolones are used as treatment. Although the bacterium can survive for many months, it is susceptible to appropriate disinfectants.

Salmonella Paratyphoid

This salmonella bacteria is capable of causing enteritis and septicaemia in young poults. Transmission may be through shell contamination, but once established it can remain in the local environment and in any rodent population. The infection is spread by faeces, fomites and poorly stored contaminated feed. Birds more readily succumb to the disease if they are not on a balanced diet, have been chilled, do not have adequate fresh water supply or already have a bacterial infection. They will have ruffled feathers, closed eyes, diarrhoea, vent pasting, will lose their appetite and look thoroughly dejected. Treatment is through Tetracycline, Amoxycillin or Fluoroquinolones. Thoroughly disinfect housing, feeders, drinkers etc. and make certain that feed is stored in a clean, dry and wild bird and rodent free area.

Salmonella Typhimurium and Enteritidis

These are the salmonella bacteria often associated with human food poisoning, so it is important to always consider personal hygiene and wash hands thoroughly after cleaning out or handling birds. The signs of disease and predisposing factors of disease are similar to those of salmonella paratyphoid. The bacteria generally live in the intestines and can be carried by contact with infected faeces, fomites and contaminated eggshells. Vertical transmission is through infected breeders via contamination of the egg yolk or through eggshell contamination. The bacteria survives successfully in the environment but can be controlled by suitably concentrated disinfectants. Treatment is the same as for salmonella paratyphoid and good hygiene and management is essential for control and prevention of the disease. This should also include the control of vermin and prevention of contamination from wild birds.

Thrush (Monialiasis)

This disease, also called sour crop, is caused by Monilia fungi and can be extremely debilitating to the bird as it grows, primarily in the crop, but it can also be found in the mouth and gizzard. It is a yeast and takes the form of tiny cream coloured ulcers that, together, look like a mass of curds and can, over time, completely line the crop. It is one of those diseases that is not obviously noticeable, but an affected turkey will become listless and lose its appetite along with loss of weight, espe-

cially on the chest. Although the effects can be quite dramatic, it is a disease that can only be confirmed on post-mortem. Thrush is another diseases which arises as a result of unhygienic conditions, mainly in equipment. Treatment is difficult because the fungus will 'feed' on antibiotics, so these should not be administered. Nystatin is worth trying.

Transmissible Enteritis – Bluecomb

Bluecomb in turkeys is a viral disease that was first recognised in America in 1944 amongst birds on muddy ranges. It may be coincidental that the pasture was muddy, but it is certainly known that mud harbours healthcare problems, so these conditions should be avoided if at all possible. Bluecomb can affect a complete group of turkeys at once and the mortality rate varies from very few to all. Transmission is through infected birds or faeces. The turkeys become anorexic, depressed and their body temperature falls, so they huddle together for warmth. The head darkens, crops are sour and they pass loose brownish droppings. It is treated with antibiotics. Both Terramycin or Aureomycin are affective. You must also keep the birds warm and their litter clean.

Tumours

Unfortunately, as in all other animals, turkeys can be affected by tumours, ie. lumps and bumps. Although there are several diseases that can manifest associated symptoms, if these possibilities can be ruled out with treatments it may come down to the presumption that illness could be caused by a tumour. If a turkey appears to be quite healthy and then exhibits an inability to stand without wobbling, it could well be that a tumour affecting the spinal chord could be the problem. Symptoms will probably depend on where the tumour is located, but loss of weight or simply a miserable bird may be the first you know. Sadly this is usually when the tumour has grown quite a bit and damaged organs, so the prognosis will inevitably be very poor. A veterinary surgeon will do everything possible to eliminate other illnesses, eventually treating it with steroid injections, but if the bird continues to decline it will be in its own interest to put it to sleep.

Turkey Coryza

This is a respiratory disease associated with Bordetella avium. It causes a loss of voice, eye and nasal discharge, snick (sneezing), failing appetite and difficulty breathing. Antibiotics do little to treat this disease, so a clean environment with good ventilation for the birds is essential. Good drinking water hygiene is necessary and soluble vitamins or poultry tonic in the water will aid recuperation.

Turkey Rhinotracheitis (TRT)

A disease of turkeys caused by the pneumovirus genus Paramyxoviridae, this can be passed from bird to bird but can also be transmitted by fomites. Failing appetite, loss of voice, swollen sinuses, nasal and eye discharge and swollen heads are typical signs, especially in young birds. Adult birds also produce thin-shelled and depigmented eggs. Antibiotics are not effective, so make sure the birds are in a clean, dry and dust-free environment, with fresh multivitamin drinking water. It is possible to vaccinate against TRT but if only a few turkeys are kept and their environment is hygienic it should not be necessary.

Turkey Viral Hepatitis

An unidentified virus causes this infection in turkeys. It brings about depression and occasional death in birds which appear to be in an otherwise good condition. During post-mortem analysis haemorrhaging may be seen. There is no treatment, but with good husbandry many birds do recover. Turkey viral hepatitis is another disease that should not manifest itself if the birds are kept in a clean, dry and dust-free environment.

Worms

Just like cats, dogs and other animals, turkeys can become infested with worms and they should routinely be treated. There are various types that live in different parts of the body.

Ascaridia Dissimilis (Roundworm)

Roundworm is the most common and can be a serious threat. Although there may only be a few adult worms in a turkey's intestines, from these will develop numerous larvae, which will have a significant effect on the bird's health. Birds may just be unthrifty or may lay smaller eggs. Roundworms can cause a necrotic-like enteritis and subsequent E.coli infection as well as migrating to other parts, in particular the liver and causing damage. A severe infestation of roundworms can block the intestines, even causing them to rupture and may be visible in the bird's droppings.

Capillaria Contorta (Hairworm)

Hairworm is a thin, hair-like pale coloured roundworm anything from 7 to 18mm in length that infests the crop and oesophagus. Capillaria obsignata is found in the small intestine. Infection is through the oral route. These worms, although small, can do a lot of damage and can be very debilitating to the affected birds.

Cestodes (Tapeworm)

Tapeworm is a segmented parasitic worm which attaches to the small intestine by its head. Growth is from the head outwards, so the segments furthest from the head are the ripest and contain the eggs. These segments containing the eggs will break away and eventually be passed out of the turkey's body via the droppings. The minute eggs are then ingested by a smaller being such as an insect, slug or earthworm, whereupon they hatch. The turkey then becomes infected when it eats the insect that contains the tapeworm cyst. There are many different species of tapeworm to which turkeys are host and these can vary from minuscule worms to some around 25cm (10 inches) in length. All too often you won't even know that your birds have tapeworms.

Heterakis Gallunarum (Caecal worm)

This is a nematode parasitic worm up to 1.5cm in length that is found in the caecum. It causes inflammation of the caecum, but more importantly it can carry another parasite, Histomonas meleagridis, which causes Blackhead.

Histomonas (Blackhead)

Blackhead is the disease of most concern to turkey keepers and more often than not it is fatal. Histomonas meleagridis is a protozoan parasite which chickens can carry, but turkeys, pheasants, game birds and peafowl are the most susceptible. The parasite is ingested in the ova of heterakis worms or as larvae in earthworms and the incubation period is fifteen to twenty days. The main sign of blackhead is a sulphur yellow diarrhoea, depression with head sunk into shoulders, a lack of appetite and emaciation. The parasite attacks the liver, which is why the condition is often fatal.

It is difficult to cure as the drug which has in the past been successful in dealing with this disease, Dimetridazole, has been banned from use in the European Union. Metronidazole is now used in the form of Flagyl tablets. Another product which can be useful in treating birds with blackhead is Stomorgy 110 which contains Metronidazole plus Spiromycin. Good hygiene and fresh pasture help to prevent blackhead occurring. It is never a good idea to put turkeys on land which has been inhabited by chickens, especially if it has been occupied by them for a long period.

Syngamus Trachea (Gapeworm)

Gapeworm is a nematode parasitic worm which, as the name suggests, lives in the windpipe. They can infest this part of the anatomy so severely that the bird chokes, hence the 'gaping' for breath implied by the name. Infection is via the oral route, earthworms, slugs and snails being hosts, but it is also possible for a turkey to ingest the embryonated egg directly. Gapeworm is more likely to affect free range birds, especially where wild birds may be present, for instance, near a rookery.

Evidence of gapeworm infestation is seen through the bird gaping in a desperate attempt to breathe and in a heavy infestation of roundworm it may be possible to see worms that have been excreted in the faeces. Any turkey with worms will gradually lose condition, become mopey and listless and will begin to lose weight. By the time worms are really affecting the system diarrhoea will also be apparent. It is vital that turkeys are treated for worms and this should never be done on an 'only when remembered' basis! Poor condition could eventually lead to death so you will need to have in place a regular programme of worming with the aim of keeping the birds free of adult, egg laying worms. Worming may need to be as frequent as every six weeks, especially if turkeys are with chickens when all the birds need be treated and this way the life-cycle of internal parasites will be interrupted. Flubenvet is licensed by the Veterinary Medicines Directorate (VMD) for worm treatment in poultry. It comes as a powder that is mixed in with the feed and can only be purchased from a veterinary surgeon or a qualified agricultural merchant as it is a Prescription Only Medicine (POM). Dosages for most internal parasites are clearly marked on the container, however the dosage to combat tapeworm is higher and it is recommended that a veterinary surgeon is consulted and use will depend on the purpose for which the turkeys are kept. Janssen Animal Health also market Flubenvet in countries other than the UK, but the name may be slightly different. A new product launched in 2006, Solubenol, is a wormer licensed for chickens but is also effective in turkeys. It is soluble and designed to be administered in the drinking water.

Some of the biggest health challenges to turkeys are via the gut, so keep this part of the bird as free from bacteria and parasites as possible. The pH level of a turkey's gut is 4, ideal for many of the bugs that will try to invade it. By altering this level and making the gut slightly more acidic it becomes a less hospitable environment, making it more difficult for them to pass through and go on to damage vital organs. I have found that putting a little cider vinegar in the fresh drinking water each day has shown some benefit, so perhaps this is one way of helping to create a healthier gut.

When worming turkeys all litter should be cleaned away and replaced by fresh because there will be immediate re-infestation if litter or faecal material is contaminated with worm eggs. The cleaner you can keep the housing and equipment, the better chance you will have of minimising any build up of worm eggs or other bacterial infections.

General Conclusions

Contrary to the experience of some turkey keepers I have found that these birds have a great will to live and if kept as pets they will certainly put their trust in you and can display great bravery. However, every injury or disease should be assessed by the owner and the vet together and each situation dealt with according to its severity, the overall demeanour of the bird and what the owner is prepared to undertake, both financially and as a nursing commitment. For complicated surgical treatment a vet would probably refer the patient to a specialist, but even for general turkey care there are poultry vets willing to provide a general practitioner with a second opinion.

Unfortunately there will be occasions when nothing can be done to save a turkey from dying, in which case the bird must be despatched by a trained person or anaesthetised by a vet. However, if you and your veterinary surgeon have done whatever is possible to treat the problem and relieve the pain you will, as an owner, have done your best for the bird.

Veterinary medicines are regularly reviewed by the European Union Veterinary Standing Committee and more specifically the Veterinary Medicines Directorate in the UK. In time, medicines suggested in this book may be withdrawn or replaced by others. A product which is used to treat a condition in a species for which it is not authorised (licensed) is only possible if the product is prescribed by a veterinary surgeon who knows the birds involved and in circumstances where no product authorised for the conditions and species being treated is available. In this case veterinary surgeons may, on their own responsibility and with the owner's consent, prescribe for animals under their care, medicines for a use that is not in accordance with the manufacturer's authorised recommendation (off label use).

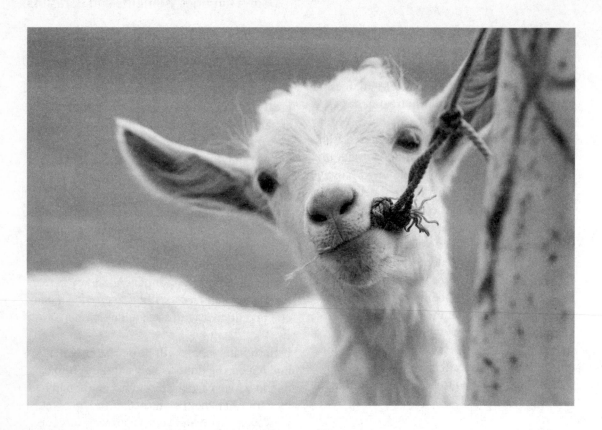

Chapter Four

PREVENTION AND EARLY DIAGNOSIS OF GOAT AILMENTS

By Felicity Stockwell

Goats have a worldwide reputation for being either very alive or very dead and not much in between! However, with careful husbandry and good practices most common ailments can be avoided, and when they do occur they can be treated by the goat keeper.

Many vets have minimal experience of goats, but it is advised to persist and find a large animal vet in your area. Sometimes an experienced goat keeper is the person to ask if you are unsure. Following or failing that, then obtaining the services of your vet must always be considered a priority and is, in fact, a legal requirement. When contemplating goat keeping, enquiring locally about a vet with some caprine experience is a worthwhile exercise.

It should be noted that many preparations are not licensed for goat use and although sheep preparations are usually eminently suitable, care should be taken and advice sought if necessary as to which to use, particularly if the goat is producing milk for human consumption or destined for the abattoir within the next 3 to 4 weeks.

From pregnancy to birth and throughout the goat's life I shall endeavour to provide an easy reference point for common problems that can be easily dealt with by the hobby goat keeper/smallholder and also a guide to when you should call for professional assistance.

A Few Basics

The normal temperature of a healthy goat is 39/39.5°C. Their heart rate should be 70 to 80 beats per minute with a normal respiration rate of 10 to 30 breaths per minute. The normal rumen activity of a healthy goat is between 1 and 1½ movements per minute.

How To Take A Temperature

Take the temperature rectally, ideally with a digital thermometer. If you use a glass thermometer make sure you shake down the mercury before use. Tie the goat up, Lubricate the end of the thermometer with a little petroleum jelly, hold the goat's tail up with one hand and gently insert the thermometer. She may initially startle (well, wouldn't you!), but will soon relax. Record the temperature for one minute or until the beeper sounds, if using a digital thermometer with this facility.

How To Take A Heart/Pulse Rate

You do not need a stethoscope for this. If you place both your hands on either side of the goat's chest behind the elbows and low down, you will be able to feel the heart rate quite clearly.

How To Use A Stethoscope

For taking heart rates and listening to rumen activity I prefer to use a stethoscope. They are easily purchased for just a few pounds. You do not need a high tech one! For taking the heart rate, apply the stethoscope to the goat on the near side, just behind the elbow. Let the heart rate settle for a few seconds as it may elevate initially. Use the second hand on your watch to establish the beat. If you are monitoring a potentially unwell animal, make a physical note of the heart rate and time taken for future comparison.

How To Check Respiration Rate

This is purely visual, although a goat that is breathing heavily can be heard. Watch the goat's nostrils and count the in and out breath. Each breath in and out again constitutes one breath and that is what you use to count.

How To Check Rumen Activity

The movement of the rumen can clearly be felt by pushing your fist firmly but gently into the goats flank, which is midway between the ribs and thigh.

Common Skin Conditions

Ringworm

Ringworm is a fungus that lives on wood and fences for years and is easily contracted. The goat needs to have only a small scratch for the fungus to enter the skin. The usual scenario is that the goat scratches on an infected post and thus introduces the fungus. It takes 10 days from introduction to signs of the first lesions. It tends to start as a small pustule that progresses to many pustules which in turn create a 'ring' of lesions, which is normally the point at which it is noticed. The goat will scratch the affected area(s), thus further infecting other areas of the goat house/field. Organic treatment consists of using freshly squeezed lemon juice on the site, initially followed by dusting with Flowers of Sulphur or applying Gentian Violet. Ringworm is self limiting and will eventually disappear on its own. However, failure to treat will cause a major and reoccurring outbreak in all your livestock. All wooden areas where the goat has rubbed should be creosoted or sprayed with Virkon S. Keep livestock away from creosote for 2 days after application.

Skin Parasites

Treat goats twice a year with a topical skin application. Pour the powder or liquid down the spine from poll to tail and it will naturally follow the hair line around the goat.

If you suspect your goat has a skin problem then examine its skin closely with a magnifying glass or at the very least your very best reading glasses! Tiny droppings or eggs from lice or mites are easily missed without assistance of this kind! You canot see mange mites without a microscope.

Mites

Mites are essentially mange mites or occasionally forage mites and the goat will bite and scratch at itself, giving rise to a patchy, woolly appearance of the coat and latterly leathery skin patches and loss of condition in a surprisingly short time. It is important to establish which mite is causing the problem and it will be necessary for your vet to take a skin scraping for microscopic investigation in order to prescribe the correct treatment. This is an urgent situation as it is highly contagious and the goat will become debilitated very quickly.

Harvest Mites

These commonly affect grazing goats and usually inhabit the area between the claws and the lower parts of the legs. They collect in clusters which show as an orangey red dot or dots. There are literally thousands of them in each 'dot' and a magnifying glass will be required to see them individually. The goat will bite at its lower legs and stamp its feet as they are intensely itchy. Treat with either tea tree oil, sulphur powder, or Spot On spray.

Lice

Lice live on the coat and skin and are just visible to the naked eye, but easily spotted with a magnifying glass! Treat with louse powder such as Delete by pouring from the poll to the tail. The preparation will work its way through the coat. Treat ALL the goats regardless of whether or not they are showing symptoms. Once treated, immediately remove them from their pens to a paddock or clean area. Remove and burn all bedding and disinfect the goat house with Virkon S. Sprinkle louse powder into the corners. Re-bed and return the goats to their house.

Worming

Wormers fall into three different categories and it is important to identify the chemicals used in each preparation and to change your wormer annually. The importance of this is to avoid wormer resistance becoming established. There is a temptation to use a variety of wormers throughout the year, but this should be avoided or resistance to several wormers can be experienced.

The three groups of wormers are as follows:
- Benzamidazoles and probenzamidazoles *(white coloured wormers eg. Panacur)*

- Levamisole *(yellow wormers eg. Levacur)*
- Avermectines *(often clear coloured eg. Oramec)*

All goats should be wormed regularly, but not over wormed as this can lead to resistance to wormers and is also expensive for you. Virtually all wormers are prepared for sheep and goats metabolise drugs quicker than sheep, so you should double the sheep dose per kilo when using wormers from the Benzamidazole and Lavamisole group and increase by 50% for Avermectines per kilo of goat weight.

Depending on your herd size, acreage grazed and space shared with other species, your goats may need a worm dosing anything from twice annually to every six weeks. Advice is best sought from your vet who will know local conditions and will be able to advise accordingly as every situation will be different. Having a worm count done once or twice a year is also a good plan. The cost is small compared to the wasteful use of wormer. You can use your veterinary practice for this or a number of direct testing laboratories can be found on the internet.

It is a good idea to worm a doe 2 days after kidding as there is often a rise of worms at this time.

Organic Worming

If you decide to avoid using chemical wormers a regular worm count will be essential. There are various organic wormers available that usually involve dosing over a protracted period of time. One of these is Verm X, a pelleted wormer which is added to feed. These are not always effective, but are worth trying.

Invasive Injuries

The most likely injuries that a goat is liable to sustain are from wire, broken branches, glass, biting by other goats and head injuries from other goats through butting.

Making sure that your grazing areas, pens and outbuildings are free from obvious hazards is the first port of call, Make sure that there are no nails sticking out, no bits of baler twine lying around, no broken glass or old (or new for that matter) farm machinery accessible to your goats. Keep thorn bushes trimmed back so that accidental injury cannot occur to eyes and noses. Should an invasive injury occur then bring the goat in and clean the area with saline solution. Use a large disposable syringe without a needle for this purpose as you can direct the jet into the wound to fully irrigate it. Use a magnifying glass to examine the wound carefully for any remaining foreign bodies and flush the wound further if required. If there is a gaping wound or a flap of skin larger than 3cm then a vet should be called to suture as necessary and administer antibiotics. Should the latter be necessary then your vet will almost certainly give you a 3 day supply of antibiotics which you can inject yourself. He/she will explain whether the antibiotics need to be administered subcutaneously(under the skin) or intra muscularly (into the muscle). Do not be afraid to ask how to do it if you are unsure.

Assuming that veterinary intervention is not required, you should then treat the irrigated wound with aloe vera gel and a topical wound powder. Aloe has wonderful healing properties and the wound powder will prevent flies attacking the site. Dab around the wound with fly repellent if flies are present, depending on the time of year. It would be wise to keep the goat penned for 2 or 3 days, dressing the wound once or twice daily. Once healing has begun keep an eye on the area for any signs of secondary infection such as pus, dying back of the skin or a bad smell. Any of these signs will necessitate a visit from a vet.

Biting

Female goats occasionally have a habit of attacking each others' udders with disastrous results! Usually this is caused by a group of females with kids when mis-mothering takes place or a new individual is introduced to the herd. It is something to be constantly aware of in a group of lactating females. Usually it will result only in bruising, but that bruising can be a precursor to mastitis and should always be taken seriously. The offending goat needs to be removed from the herd if this is more than an isolated incident and consideration must be given as to whether rehoming of this individual is appropriate in the long term.

Bruising can be dealt with by the application of udder ointment and hot and cold compresses. Arnica cream is also a very effective treatment and would be my own first choice. Watch out for 'hot spots' developing on the udder over the next few days as this can be a sign of mastitis developing.

Rips or tears of the udder tissue caused by biting are more serious and immediate veterinary intervention is mandatory if you are to keep your goat healthy and productive. A large milking udder has no chance of making a reasonable natural repair without help.

Occasionally ears get bitten or torn, the latter usually as a result of an ear tag getting entangled in wire netting or a hay feeder. Arnica cream is useful for bruising without broken skin and Aloe Vera for broken skin after flushing with saline. Bruised ears can often end up alarmingly swollen but, as long as there is no real heat, continued treatment with Arnica will usually resolve the problem in about a week.

Butting

Butting can happen at any time. Avoid keeping horned and hornless goats together as the horned goats are at a distinct advantage and can inflict some lethal injuries. Young males will often play fight and this is fine unless it is continued and prolonged. Anything that causes bleeding or that you can see is becoming serious should prompt you to separate the offending individuals. Treat horn bud injuries with antiseptic spray or wound powder. Keep away from other animals until healing is under way and be very careful about fly strike on these areas. Use your intelligence to work out why the problem occurred and address the management of your stock accordingly.

Lameness

Establish which foot your goat is actually lame on. It will 'drop' on the good foot and 'go light' on the bad one. A goat with a shuffley gait is probably lame on all four feet and this is likely to be caused by laminitis due to overfeeding or scald, a bacterium which thrives in grassland in temperatures consistently over 10°C and as such is very much a spring complaint.

Secure the goat and check the affected foot. Does it need trimming? Is the foot damaged, sore or bleeding? Is there anything stuck between the digits or soreness in the lower leg? Is there any swelling or heat?

Having established which one of these things it might be, take the necessary remedial action for invasive injuries, skin parasites, footrot, laminitis or trimming hooves as necessary.

Footrot And Laminitis

Footrot is a condition caused by a bacterium

and needs temperatures consistently above 10°C to proliferate. The goat has heat and swelling between the claws of the front feet and in white hoofed goats a redness will be seen around the coronet. The hoof becomes underun quite quickly and there can be separation of the horn from the sensitive laminae. As a result the goat is extremely lame and will often graze on its knees. It is mainly a condition of outdoor goats, but can be contracted by housed goats and passed on throughout the herd. It can be controlled in fields by removing the goats from the pasture for a minimum of ten days and returning them after that period of time has elapsed and the feet have been treated. Do this by dipping the feet in zinc sulphate. If this is just for a few goats it can be done by immersing the feet individually into the solution in a plastic tub or small bucket. Where there are a lot of goats a foot bath should be used. Where it is a serious and ongoing problem the goats can be vaccinated with a vaccine called Footvax. It is intended for sheep but most vets will supply it for goats.

Laminitis is the inflammation of the laminae of the goat's feet. The laminae are like little leaves of horn which overlay one another. If the goat has access to sudden high levels of protein which can typically be concentrated feed or lush spring grass, this causes these 'leaves' to become inflamed and engorged with blood, which makes the goat extremely lame and the feet hot and painful to the touch. The goat will lie down or stand with its weight on its heels. Addressing the diet and obtaining anti-inflammatory drugs from your vet are the first action. Once the goat recovers it will have a tendency to contract laminitis again, so great attention to diet is essential.

Laminitis can also be a complication of post kidding illnesses such as mastitis and metritis.

Hoof Trimming

Hoof trimming is a vital part of goat husbandry and should be undertaken every six weeks. It is particularly important in both assisting recovery and avoiding hoof conditions such as footrot and laminitis.

Use a hoof knife and/or hoof shears to trim correctly and follow up with a surform file or some coarse sandpaper. Take small slices off at a time to avoid over trimming, which can cause the hoof to bleed. If this should happen the goat will be lame for a few days, but you must treat the hoof with antibiotic spray or tea tree oil for several days to avoid infection entering the wound.

Loss Of Appetite

Goats can lose their appetite for a number of reasons. If this is the case they should be observed for the signs and symptoms of illness, poisoning and disease. It is vital that they recommence eating as soon as possible as rumen activity is vital for their survival. Initially check that food is not contaminated by the goat, other goats or other animals and check that the water supply is clean. Take the goat's temperature and other vital signs and check too whether it has diarrhoea. If these are all normal, try offering a 'favourite food' or treats such as digestive biscuits, grapes, banana, apple or willow. Occasionally a few ivy leaves or a piece of honeysuckle will get a goat going in terms of eating. Having exhausted all possibilities and if the goat has not begun to eat in four hours, your vet should be consulted.

NB. A goat on the verge of labour will often not eat for 3 or 4 hours beforehand. Providing all is progressing normally you can reintroduce light feeding after delivery.

Diarrhoea

Sudden changes in diet, poisoning, chronic worm infestation and toxin producing bacteria can all cause this problem.

Avoiding sudden feeding changes including giving gluts of any vegetables from your holding and worm regularly.

Give strict attention to the cleanliness of feeding utensils and housing and do not graze kids on land that was grazed by last year's kids (coccidiosis). Any diarrhoea that does not clear up in 24 hours should be considered an urgent veterinary problem. Your vet will undoubtedly take a sample for laboratory investigation and the goat or goats can be treated with anthelmintics (wormers), antibiotics or the appropriate medication as necessary. Vaccination with Heptavac P Plus will avoid the risk of Clostridial diseases, which can quickly kill goats.

Treat dietary diarrhoea (scour) by increasing hay and decreasing concentrates. The goat should be given a proprietory electrolyte such as Lectade according to the manufacturer's instructions or, failing that, a dessertspoon of glucose and a teaspoon of salt in approximately ½ gallon of water and given in a bucket (do not drench!). Kaolin can also be used, but consult with your vet on quantity and actual severity of the scour. If more than one of your goats has scour then this must be investigated by your vet as soon as possible.

Dietary Deficiencies

Dietary deficiencies can manifest themselves in many ways, but usually poor coat condition, low milk production and failure to breed efficiently are obvious signs. By feeding your goats a good and balanced diet and using a proprietary goat mix, most problems should be avoidable. Do not use feed which has been prepared for other species, particularly sheep. Sheep feed does not contain copper and goats need copper. As standard your goats should have access to a caprine salt/mineral lick and, if possible, a good vitamin/mineral supplement such as Caprivite. Check with your local vet what deficiencies your local soil may have and take advice as to how to correct these. As a general rule, the UK is deficient in both selenium and cobalt and so a combination of hanging a 'Rockie Red' block which has added copper and a 'Rockie SC Sheep' block will provide the selenium and cobalt. Any goat showing signs of unthriftiness should be blood tested by your vet to eliminate any serious notifiable problems such as Caprine Arthritis Encephalitis (CAE), TB (identified in goats in the UK for the first time in many years in 2008), Scrapie and Johne's disease.

Fibre goats (Angora, Cashmere/Cashgora) need to have a higher protein level in their diets than other goats. They need to be fed the same as a lactating dairy doe as the growth of fleece takes large proportions of the goat's energy. As a result, if the dietary requirements are not met, the quality of the fleece will be lower and the goat's bodily condition will suffer. It is important to condition score a fibre goat by feeling its hindquarters for fleshiness as the coat will hide the skeletal condition. If not you may have a shock when the goat is shorn. Additional sulphur is also required by fibre goats and this can be achieved by feeding one ounce of Sulphur Sublimed per animal per week, mixed through the weekly ration. Sulphur Sublimed, also known as Flowers of Sulphur, is an acrid yellow powder. If it is any other colour you have the wrong kind of sulphur, so don't use it! Alternatively you can supplement the diet with an Angora specific supplement such as Caprivite Angora.

Poisoning

Unlike most livestock, goats seem to have a knack of finding all the food that poisons them! Great care must be taken when collecting browsings or turning a goat out onto pasture that there is nothing growing in hedges and on stone walls that might poison them. Certain plants will poison a goat quickly and create a problem from which it is unlikely to recover. Generally speaking, if a goat has a full rumen, ingestion of small quantities of poisonous plants have a lesser effect but plant poisoning in goats is totally avoidable if you are observant and careful of your goat grazing areas. Always check the perimeters and hedgerows and if your holding or field is flanked by neighbours, pay them a friendly visit and request that they do not feed your animals in any circumstances or deposit their garden debris on your boundaries.

Should your goat be unfortunate enough to ingest a poisonous plant or substance, this is an emergency situation. If possible ascertain the cause of the poisoning and call your vet immediately.

Routine Vaccination And Administration

Vaccination of goats is not considered essential by some, but my personal feelings are that it is essential!

Bluetongue

The use of Bluetongue vaccine (currently BTV8) is not yet compulsory in the UK but I suspect it may become so. This vaccine can only be obtained from a vet for your own administration. Goats should receive 2 subcutaneous injections of 1ml given 4 weeks apart and followed by six monthly boosters. Kids can be vaccinated at four weeks old using vaccine produced by Intervet and at 3 months old with vaccine produced by Merriel. Bottles of vaccine must be used within eight hours of opening and contain a minimum of 20 doses, so for small scale keeping, obtaining syringes of vaccine from your vet if you only have two or three goats to vaccinate makes economic sense. (Of course, if you have cows or sheep as well you could use a full bottle on each occasion.) Your vet will usually time the opening of a bottle with the needs of several other small scale keepers and so it will be necessary to speak to the surgery in advance. Once on the 'list' most practices will contact you just prior to your vaccine requirement to find out how many doses you require. The cost will be about £1 per dose, a small price to pay to protect both yours and the wider National Flock. Smallholders often get blamed for the spread of disease so we should be especially vigilant that we get it right! Bluetongue is a very real and potentially catastrophic disease.

Tetanus and Clostridial Vaccine

Tetanus is vital (for you too, but go to your Doctor!) and goats should be vaccinated every six months by using Heptavac P Plus vaccine which covers tetanus and all the clostridial diseases, some of which are transmissible to man so really shouldn't be ignored.

This vaccine should be given as a primary course of two injections given 4 to 6 weeks apart. Give 2ml subcutaneously to each goat with a six monthly 2ml booster. It can be given to kids from 2 weeks old, but if the pregnant doe has received a booster 2 to 4 weeks before she has kidded, then vaccination of the kids can be deferred until 10 weeks of age. Vaccinate all kids, even if they are destined for the freezer.

Remember that no vaccines should be given closer than 2 weeks apart so you will need to work out a regime to make sure that your boosters fall at the right time of the year and don't clash with the bluetongue vaccination which needs to be done ideally in February and August to coincide with the rise of mosquitoes and midges.

How To Keep It Clean

The importance of keeping an opened bottle of vaccine hygienic throughout the vaccination process cannot be emphasised enough. Abscesses can form very easily on a goat through bad hygiene which can lead to pain, infection and spoilage of the goat's appearance or skin if it is destined for meat and skin production.

Use one needle for withdrawal of the vaccine from the bottle, leave in situ and attach the syringe to a new needle. Use a new needle for each goat. You can use the withdrawal needle for the last goat you vaccinate.

A subcutaneous injection means beneath the skin. The best way to ensure that the vaccine goes below the skin and not into a muscle or blood vessel is to take a pinch of skin (like a tent) and push the needle into it, making sure that the needle doesn't reappear out the other side! Using a needle of the correct length is also vital. If you feel more comfortable cleaning the area with surgical spirit first then by all means do so, but if your goats are clean, kept in clean conditions and you use a separate needle for each animal, this won't be necessary.

An intramuscular injection means into the muscle. A large muscle mass needs to be chosen either in the hindquarters or the shoulder. With someone holding the goat if possible or, if not, after tying it up, gently but firmly 'prime' the area with the heel of your clenched fist.

When The End Is Inevitable …and The Law

The worst decision that any livestock keeper has to make is undoubtedly to take a life.

Some of your goats may already be destined for the freezer and so that mindset is already established and is easier to deal with, but sometimes we have to make decisions of another kind because a goat is very sick, very old or unthrifty. As humans we have the ability to end the suffering of animals and must realise that whatever our thought processes are, animals do not understand them and nor do they understand the concept of being killed. If we are very ill or in pain, we know that in the passage of time things will change. An animal doesn't know that. For all animals, suffering is the here and the now and is something they must endure until it becomes unendurable. We can change that and must recognise when that is the case.

Goats going to an abattoir for human consumption will be stunned like sheep and will have their throats cut whilst unconscious and be bled to death. That is what happens to goats and sheep - like it or not. If you cannot bear that thought, have unwanted kids put down at birth by humane injection by your vet. Alternatively you can rear them kindly and with compassion and go with them to a small local abattoir (if one exists), having prearranged the visit to be at a 'quiet' time so that they can be despatched quickly and you can see the carcasses before you leave, or in some cases you will be allowed to watch the process if you wish. This way you will satisfy yourself that all was done well and humanely. Never ever sell your kids to someone for meat unless you are personally acquainted with them and know their methods and facilities. How often have I heard, "Oh, they went to the man that takes all the unwanted kids." You might be lucky but your goats may end up the victims of ritual slaughter or worse.

Goats that have reached the end of their 'working' lives and cannot be kept as companion animals or who are unthrifty or terminally sick should be humanely despatched by your vet by lethal injection if possible. Your local knacker man is also a possibility. Make sure you have their contact details in a safe place or on your mobile phone for emergencies. These people are expert in what they do. They do an awful lot of it and it is quick and skilled as the goat is shot through the head and literally drops where it stands. The advantage of the knacker man is that they will take the carcass away. If the goat is put down by a vet by shooting or lethal injection you will have to deal with the disposal which will mean a collection for incineration or delivery of the dead goat by yourself to the nearest animal crematorium. The cost of this varies, but may range from thirty to a hundred pounds.

A goat, regardless of status, even if it is a pet or a pygmy, is an agricultural animal and must be disposed of correctly and legally. You cannot under any circumstances bury it on your own land, although you may bury the legally cremated remains.

Inevitably, if you are a stock keeper, sooner or later you are going to be faced with these problems, so having a contingency plan in place and sticking to it is an essential part of compassionate small scale farming.

Organic Or Otherwise?

In a bid to be organic, or shall we say chemical free, there are a number of homeopathic options for caring for your goats. My own first aid kit for goats includes many organic remedies, but if you want or need to be totally purist for personal or legal reasons, perhaps because you are organically registered, then taking advice from your Organic Status Provider is essential and perhaps enlist the services of a homeopathic vet.

Pregnancy And Birth

Your goat will have a pregnancy of approximately 151 days, but a variation of four or five days on either side is normal, so be prepared! Regardless of category type she will have been mated by a buck or buckling (NB. male kids are fertile from 16 weeks of age, so be aware of this to avoid any stolen matings!) any time from July to March, which is the normal cycle time for goats in the Northern Hemisphere. Most goats will be mated in the Autumn with a view to a spring kidding when herbage is actively growing again. This will ensure a plentiful supply of grass for the mother and ultimately the kids who will start to graze and pick at around ten days old.

The most common problems of pregnancy are:

Abortion

This can be caused by infection or by some abnormality in the foetus.

The first thing you will notice is a discharge from the goat well before her kidding date - perhaps between 30 and 140 days - and at this point you should isolate her from the other goats and keep an eye on her. If she appears to be well in herself, then it is a waiting game. If she seems unwell call your vet immediately. Over a period of time, which should not be more than twelve hours, she will abort the foetus and placenta. Wearing rubber gloves you should deposit the whole thing in a plastic bag for further examination to find the cause of the problem. Contact your vet so that tests can be carried out and perhaps a blood test from the doe (female/nanny). Remember that, although spontaneous abortion can be non-infectious, there are around 10 different serious organisms that can cause infectious abortion and these are contractable by other goats and, in some cases, humans, so personal hygiene is absolutely essential. Whatever the outcome the goat's pen must be thoroughly cleaned and sprayed with a preparation such as Virkon S which is available from vets or agricultural merchants nationwide. Clean the goat's rear end with a mild shampoo and warm water and return her to the clean, dry and freshly bedded pen. Feed plenty of hay and green food as available. Within a few days she will be ready to rejoin her companions and results should be in from your vet as to what the cause was and appropriate action can then be taken as required.

Cloudburst

This is a false pregnancy of the goat and she, you and her body will be equally convinced that she is pregnant. She will make up gallons of amniotic fluid, probably go to term and then produce….a lot of water! The downside is no kid, the upside is that she will probably come into milk as normal, can be mated again and may never experience a repeat of the problem. Although considered reasonably rare, I have experienced this situation twice in one year. There is nothing you can do on this one. It is not so much an ailment as a situation and the goat will almost certainly go on to produce healthy kids in subsequent pregnancies.

Pregnancy Toxaemia

A metabolic disease which will require veterinary intervention, but speed of recognition by the keeper is the key to the goat's survival. It will generally occur when the goat is fed inappropriately for its stage of pregnancy and

occurs towards the end of pregnancy, typically in the last 2 weeks. Her breath will have a sweet smell (peardrops) and she may grind her teeth, be off her food altogether and, worse still, become prone and reluctant to rise. This is an urgent situation and the vet must be called to administer drugs which may help to reverse the release of ketones in her blood which is causing this. At best she will deliver her kids early, which may or may not survive. With luck she will recover but, at worst, left untreated, she will become prone, then die within 6 or 7 days.

Toxaemia of pregnancy can be avoided by feeding plenty of good quality forage in the last 8 weeks of pregnancy and lower quantities of concentrates (typically no more than 1kg per day for a dairy goat, 500g for a fibre goat and 250g for a pygmy goat), by ensuring daily exercise, by avoiding trauma and stress during the last couple of weeks of pregnancy and by avoiding mating overweight goats.

Kidding

Approximately two weeks before the expected date of kidding the doe should be established in her kidding pen. If she is free range with access to a shelter (a must for all goats) it is possible to create a corner for her using sheep hurdles and screening them with straw bales. Clean out all old bedding and disinfect solid floors and walls or use a preparation such as Stalosan disinfectant powder if the structure is of an organic nature. Keep her warm and draft free and allow her out during the day if the weather allows.

Her concentrate ration should be kept low at no more than 0.5kg per day, but she should be given ad lib forage (hay/straw) which should be fed above ground, preferably in a hayrack. The importance of acclimatising her to a confined area is to allow her to build up colostral antibodies which she will pass on to her kids to keep them safe in those first few days after birth. Make sure that you have your own kidding kit which should contain the following essential equipment:

- A new bar of soap and nail brush
- A pair of nail scissors
- Iodine or coloured antiseptic spray
- Your vet's telephone number
- Clean towels
- A pair of clean waterproof over trousers
- Obstetric lubricating gel and long armed examination gloves (optional)

Imminent Kidding

The signs of imminent kidding are:

A full udder (although she may have bagged up several days earlier). However full that udder is, do not, under any circumstances, milk anything off. It's early contents are colostrum, which is a vital first boost to the newborn kids for the first few days of life.

A swollen vulva which becomes elongated and slack and a desire to stay in her pen that morning.

Hollows will appear at the base of her tail and she will elevate her tail in a hooked fashion.

She will circle her pen with increasing regularity and dig her bedding up (another good reason for a clean pen!). It is a good idea to give her plenty of clean straw while she continues with this, which could go on for several hours. Make sure she has a supply of clean hay, although she will only pick at it, if at all. Put her water bucket high enough so that she can drink from it, but not so low that there is any chance of her dropping a kid into it. As with humans, although there is a pattern to labour, the time the various stages take varies

hugely from person to person/goat to goat, so there are no hard and fast rules as to how long this procedure will take. In my experience, first staging can take from two to twelve hours, so don't get too excited too early if this is your first birthing or you will be exhausted by the end when you perhaps might need your wits about you.

The goat will manage this stage of labour very nicely on her own and the best thing you can do is to get on with your other jobs and check on her every 30 minutes or so. You will know when things are progressing as she will have a mucous discharge and her breathing will become more rapid with a typical flare to her nostrils. Offer her some warm water to drink. This is often appreciated, but don't worry if she is not interested. Keep strangers away from her. Whilst she will appreciate her owner's quiet attention, she will definitely not appreciate the next door neighbour's children or yours or other people's dogs. Remember that abnormal disturbance can protract the labour and possibly jeopardise an otherwise safe and successful kidding.

She will often lie down if she feels secure (I have never yet had one of my goats kid whilst standing) and usually gets this sort of 'far away' look of super concentration and shortly after you will see her strain a couple of times and the water bag will appear. In first kidders this can often retract once or twice before it stays firmly outside or just within the vulva. She may 'talk' to her unborn kids by gently bleating to them in utero – she may have been doing this for some minutes or in some cases an hour or more. Unfortunately you simply can't generalise on this subject. Quite quickly you will be able to see a little nose within the water bag or a nose and two hooves. If this is the case, don't worry. Don't interfere, all is going 100% OK! Sit quietly and watch. Don't attempt to break the water bag (membrane), the efforts of the contractions and the kid will do this perfectly well. If you break the membrane it could slow down the birth and put the kid at risk. You know that you have at least one kid arriving normally. Get your over-trousers on because you are going to get wet. Cut your nails as short as possible and wash your hands with the soap and scrub your nails with the nail brush. Keep the water because you may have to do this again if intervention is required with a subsequent kid. Alternatively you can use long armed examination gloves which can be purchased from any agricultural merchant. Assuming all is going well (and we'll deal with the negatives next) 2 or 3 good pushes by the doe should expel the kid into the world. She may shout as the head appears, but don't worry, that is quite normal.

In order to give the best assistance to your goat, get down on your knees to her level and help the doe out by pulling away the membrane, especially around the kid's nose and mouth - he will snort and splutter and shake his head - and give the goat her baby to clean up. Let her do it as the licking stimulates the kid into action and bonds mother and kid. While she is doing it she will hardly notice any further contractions and the next kid being born. Follow the same procedure with the next kid and then let the doe get on with the job for a while. If she has had a multiple birth the towel can be very useful to give her a bit of a hand with the drying process, but always let her lick her kid before you come in with the towel. Her contractions will continue and after a while the placenta will appear. She will have got to her feet by now and gravity will help her expel the placenta. Do not, under any circumstances, pull the placenta away. She must, and will, expel this on her own. I always keep some iodine or purple spray to hand which can now be used to spray the point where the umbilical cord has broken off (the cord stump). Although this is not essential if your conditions are clean, it is a wise precaution to avoid infection later and perhaps an unsightly umbilical hernia.

The 'Difficult' Kidding

I estimate from my own statistics that one in thirty kiddings is less than straightforward, but we must be mentally prepared for the worst and hopefully cope with the problems as they present themselves. It is really a question of common sense and you are a very unlucky goatkeeper if you get an insurmountable one. So what are these problems likely to be? Abnormal presentations are the most common, closely followed by the oversized kid and, last and rarely, conditions such as Ringwomb, which is a failure of the cervix to dilate and twisting or torsion of the uterus. Thankfully the latter two are uncommon, but we will touch upon them as a point of reference.

Kids coming backwards, ie. hind legs first, are quite common and seldom cause a problem unless the kid is very large. Sometimes one foreleg is back and you will see this quite clearly when a nose and a hoof appear with a second hoof not visible. Head back is another, somewhat more complicated situation and twins jammed at the pelvis are worse. This is where confidence and the bucket of hot water and soap come in again! Wash your hands again and then re-soap them or use your long armed gloves. Soap can be substituted by lubricating gel obtainable from agricultural merchant. Put all your finger tips and thumb together and very gently slide your hand into the birth canal, following the line of the goats back with the back of your hand uppermost. By the time your hand is in beyond your wrist you should be able to feel what the problem is by gently rotating your hand around until you feel the retracted limb in the case of a foreleg back or a tail in the case of a breach presentation. In the case of a foreleg back, gently grasp the hoof and pull it forward, keeping your hand over the hoof. This should bring almost immediate relief to the doe and the kid will be expelled really quickly. Help her out now to get the kid going. With a hindlegs first presentation it is probably a game of patience. The kid will almost certainly be born normally, but it will take a little longer. On no account pull a kid out; wait for a contraction and ease the kid out as an aid to each contraction, pulling downward once the head and feet or rump are clearly visible.

For a head back presentation follow the same procedure, but cradle the head in your hand and rotate it into position. Again a rapid resolution should follow.

In the case of twins jammed at the pelvis, the goat will have been straining for a good while with no results. Unless you have had significant experience it is time to get assistance from an experienced goat keeper or vet. Remember that your vet may not arrive for some time and so your main job is to stay with the mother and help as much as you can. She may be shouting a lot because she will be in pain, but if you keep calm this will help her get through the situation until help arrives.

The general rule of thumb is that if you are not sure what you can feel, the goat has been straining for an hour with no results or is becoming distressed, call for help. It is also a sensible precaution to get your vet to check any goat that has had any kind of compromised birth that has required intervention. She may need antibiotics and your vet may need to check that she has no dead kids remaining inside and that she has 'cleansed' (got rid of her placenta) properly. Never underestimate the importance of this. Far better a small vet's bill than the ramifications of a dead goat and kids and the consequences and costs of disposal. If your goat does require manual intervention at kidding she will also require antibiotic treatment from the vet.

Post Kidding

If you have more than one goat, keep the mother and newborns separate from the other goats for at least 24 hours. Make sure that the kids are feeding properly from the udder. They will always tend to favour one side in the first few days, so check that each kid has a full tummy by feeling the abdomen. If there is an excess of colostrum on one side of the udder, then utilise this by stripping some out into a sterilised bottle and freezing it for that occasion when colostrum for a weak or orphaned kid can be a lifesaver. It keeps for several years in a freezer. Very occasionally a small kid will need help to find the udder and help may be given. Once it has suckled there is usually no further problem. I always try to make sure my kids have had a feed within two hours of birth. I avoid tubing kids unless absolutely necessary - i.e. if they are unable to suck at all. Many veterinary manuals recommend this but unless you are well practised there is a risk that the kid can inhale fluids and develop pneumonia.

After kidding the mother will benefit from some warm water and a feed of sloppy oatmeal or bran with a tablespoon of honey and a pinch of salt. Resist the temptation to give her a great big scoop of concentrates! Just make sure she has plenty of good quality hay and straw in her pen again. She will eat the afterbirth once dispelled. This will not hurt her and will probably give her a boost of the right sort of protein and iron. Some goat keepers will not agree with this, but I have never had a problem and it is, after all, what nature intended. Failing that, you are really supposed to dispose of it according to Defra Rules, which means it must be incinerated. The important thing is that if the kids are born dead, malformed or the foetus is aborted before the end of the usual gestation period, then this is a much more serious matter and you should call your Animal Health Office or the Defra helpline for guidance.

Depending on the time of year, green food is always appreciated and bananas and dates are also a luxury treat which will be readily eaten.

If you have more than one goat to kid in reasonably quick succession it is a good idea to identify the kids with a coloured spray to correspond with the same colour mark on their mother. If you don't have a coloured spray then mark the ears with a coloured felt tip marker instead.

When the kids are a day old check that the females have no teat abnormalities and book your vet for disbudding at between 4 and 10 days, depending on your vet's normal practice. It is illegal in the UK to disbud kids without an anaesthetic and this must be administered by a vet. Also check for problems with the navel. Consider the use of Enterotoxaemia vaccine (Heptavac P) at 2 weeks for kids from unvaccinated mothers or at 12 weeks from vaccinated mothers.

Post Kidding Problems

Acetonaemia (Ketosis)

The symptoms of Ketosis are very similar to those of pregnancy toxaemia, but the time scale is different as Ketosis, when it occurs, is almost always a problem after delivery. It is caused by insufficient energy food in or around the fourth to sixth week post kidding as this is when the demands on her milk are going to be highest, particularly if she has kids at foot. The doe's breath will smell sweet, not dissimilar to peardrops (acetone) and she will avoid eating concentrates completely. Feed-

ing little and often is the key. If she is housed then she should be receiving the very best hay possible and/or haylage which is intended for horses (preferably a ryegrass variety). She should be allowed this ad lib and if the time of year allows, suitable harvested browsings. Her concentrate ration should be increased post kidding over four weeks and, if possible, fed in 3 out of four feeds a day, but never in one go. Depending on the breed, and assuming that you are using a proprietory goat mix, follow the manufacturer's feeding instructions with regard to quantities.

Although it is possible to help with the condition yourself, my advice would be to call your vet immediately who will be able to administer intravenous dextrose. This is something you cannot do yourself. The important thing is to make sure you can recognise the condition and act accordingly.

Mastitis

Mastitis is a problem that unfortunately once established tends to revisit on regular occasions. It is relatively unusual for a goat rearing its own offspring and that is not milked to develop mastitis. It can be caused by bruising to the teats and udder as well as bacterial infection.

Relief can be brought to the goat initially by applying hot (but not boiling) cloths to the affected area. This can often help release the congestion and allow you to milk off the milk which is known as 'beestings.' This is because it is stringy and solid and will leave the teat in clots. Antibiotic treatment may also be necessary. A goat that is known to have suffered mastitis in previous years should be managed carefully in every lactation in order to maintain usefulness as a milker. Refer chronic cases to your vet for antibiotic therapy.

Essential First Aid And Veterinary Kit For All Goat Keepers

- Thermometer
- Stethoscope
- Hand washing gel/alcohol
- Several pairs of well fitting disposable rubber gloves
- Povodine iodine concentrate
- Saline solution *(homemade is fine in a sterilised container)*
- Lubricating gel/petroleum jelly
- Virkon S sachets *(for disinfecting stalls and utensils)*
- Syringes *(disposable or re-useable)*
- Needles (½" for kids and ¾" for adults)
- An empty, sterilised washing up liquid bottle and an 8" silicone tube *(to fit nozzle for drenching)*
- Large disposable syringe for wound dressing
- Ditto for wormer
- Magnifying glass
- Aloe Vera gel or spray
- Arnica cream
- Wound powder(something suitable for horses is fine)
- Lectade electrolyte solution or powder
- Organic antiparasitic powder such as 'Delete' or chemical spray or pour-on such as Spot-On.
- Fly spray
- Mint udder cream
- BTV8 vaccine *(must be used or disposed of within 8 hours of opening and refrigerated before opening. Best obtained by the syringe from your vet if only a few animals to vaccinate)*
- Heptavac P vaccine*(observe storage guidance)*
- Wormer type *(see worming)*
- Sharp round ended scissors
- Garden sprayer *(for economic disinfection of pens, utensils and surrounding woodwork-kept specifically for the purpose)*
- Clean lidded bucket *(for veterinary use only)*

Isolation And Quarantine

If isolation of a goat is necessary for the safety of other animals try, if possible, to put the goat within eye and ear shot of other goats as they can become more distressed by being taken away from their companions.

When purchasing new stock, keeping them quarantined for 10 days is a good idea. It also gives existing goats time to become familiar with the sight of them. Make sure there is no nose to nose contact or sharing or air space, so a shed or pen within eye and ear shot of existing goats is ideal, but where physical contact between them is not possible. Wear rubber gloves when working with new goats and remove them before attending to your existing ones. Do not share drinking or feeding vessels. This may seem a little extreme but it will be well worth it if your new acquisitions show signs of disease during the days they are quarantined, which can turn into a very expensive problem if you have a lot of goats.

Utilise the time in quarantine to worm and start a vaccination programme. Only accept that the goat has been vaccinated if you have seen documentary evidence.

Twenty Ways To Avoid Accidents, Injury And Disease

1. Feed ad lib high fibre forage at all times ie. hay, haylage (but not silage) and use the best quality feed, forage and bedding you can.
2. Check for poisonous plants, trees and shrubs wherever the goats have access.
3. Avoid sudden changes of diet or increases in certain parts of it because you may have a glut of certain foods on your holding.
4. Worm and vaccinate regularly and keep accurate records of same - both are a legal and essential husbandry requirement.

5. Treat for skin parasites at least twice a year, depending on your choice of preparation.

6. Creosote fence posts and gates to avoid fungal spores remaining on them.

7. Thoroughly disinfect all pens, hurdles, drinking vessels and feed buckets, walls and floors at least once a year with Virkon S in a garden sprayer, having thoroughly cleaned out and swept the accommodation first. Allow to dry and re-bed before allowing goats back in.

8. Trim hooves every six weeks.

9. Change drinking water twice daily and scrub troughs and drinkers weekly.

10. Always feed and milk goats at the same times each day.

11. Always disinfect pens when changing goats over.

12. Quarantine new animals for 10 days.

13. Never kid a goat in a pen where other goats have kidded previously without thorough cleansing. it.

14. Do not turn out kids on an area where the previous year's kids or lambs have grazed to avoid coccidiosis infection.

15. Check your goats at least twice daily.

16. Always keep more than one goat. A single goat is a vulnerable one and more likely to succumb to disease than those kept with companions.

17. Be cautious about leaving collars on your goats, particularly if they are free range. Because of their browsing techniques it can be very easy for a goat to become entangled in branches and strangle itself. If required, sheep collars which are wide and close fitting can be employed. They will break with tension, whereas a webbing or leather collar is less likely to do so.

18. Never tether a goat, however 'hi-tech' you think your methods are! At one time the tethering of goats was almost the norm in the UK, but deaths through strangulation, broken limbs, hunger and thirst have proved that this is a totally unacceptable option and in certain circumstances is actually illegal.

19. Always accurately complete your Animal Medicine Record Book after each and every treatment, identifying the goats by name and number. It is an essential point of reference and is also required by law.

20. Avoid stress in handling, penning or moving goats.

In the UK it is a criminal offence not to deal with sick livestock in a timely and appropriate manner, summoning professional help if required. Good nursing is the key to recovery. Your own good nursing of the sick or compromised animal is probably the most important thing you will ever do for your goat. You will know that it is a sensitive, intelligent creature that entrusts itself to its keeper. Moral support, determination and constant attention can sometimes be the difference between life and death. Talk constantly and quietly to your ailing/recovering goat and leave a radio on quietly playing classical music if possible. Leave a safe nightlight on during darkness. Offer tepid water with a teaspoonful of salt to every 5 litres to encourage drinking. Pick grass and other foliage and offer it regularly to the goat. Remove anything that isn't eaten after 12 hours. Young dock leaves are often enjoyed and willow twigs and leaves.

Never be frightened to summon help if in any doubt about your own diagnosis of a problem: the loss and financial consequences of disposal and re-stocking will always be far greater than the vet's bill.

DIAGNOSTIC GUIDE TO GOAT AILMENTS AND TREATMENT

Signs of Disease	Causes	Treatment And Prevention
HEAD AND FACE		
Nasal Discharge.	Pneumonia due to virus or bacterial infection.	Antibiotic for most cases. If animal is kept indoors check ventilation.
	Most common infection is due to Pasteurella species.	Vaccine available for Pasteurella control.
	Bacterial or fungal infection in upper respiratory tract.	Antibiotic or antifungal preparations after swabbing to make diagnosis.
Ulcers on lips, tongue and dental pad.	Foot and Mouth disease (NB. notifiable disease).	Check for other symptoms eg. blisters around feet.
Scabs on lips, also on nostrils and eye lids.	Orf ie. infection by Paravaccinia virus.	Topical ointments and sprays can stop secondary bacterial infection. Isolate affected animals. Vaccine available.
Scabs on face ie. around eyes, ears and base of horn.	Facial eczema due to bacterial infection ie. Staphylococcus aureus. Not common but may be complicated by fly worry.	Antibiotic and check to make sure trough space is adequate. Insecticides can be used and head protected by head cap.
Loss of hair on face, especially around the eyes.	Ringworm, usually due to Trichophyton verrucosum. Rare condition but more common than in sheep (NB infectious to people).	Topical antifungal agents.
Salivation and drooling from the mouth.	Viral infection eg. Orf or Foot and Mouth (NB. FMD notifiable disease).	See above.
	Actinobacillosis ie. bacterial infection in the mouth and jaw bone and elsewhere.	Antibiotic or sodium iodide intravenous weekly or potassium iodide orally daily.
	Consider the possibility of foreign body stuck in mouth eg. thorn or bramble.	Have a good look with torch and mouth gag.
Swelling of lips and tongue, tongue blue in appearance.	Bluetongue (NB. notifiable disease).	Vaccinate and try to control biting flies and midges. No effective treatment.
Watery discharge from one or both eyes.	Entropion ie. inturned eye lid - unlikely in adult animal.	Minor surgery may be required.
White discharge from one or both eyes, sometimes with damage to the surface of the eye.	Infectious Kerato conjunctivitis due to infection by Rickettsia or Chlamydia bacteria.	Subconjunctival injection job for the vet or topical antibiotic ointment. Control is difficult. Reduce crowding and contol flies.
Discharge from one eye with or without eye damage.	Look for foreign body in the eye eg. hay seed.	Careful search required and then remove. Antibiotic ointment after removal.

Signs of Disease	Causes	Treatment and Prevention
HEAD AND FACE CONTINUED		
Swollen eye lids.	Allergic reaction.	Antihistamine or corticosteroid injections. May have to move pastures.
Eyes dull and lifeless.	Animal may be in pain or suffering from any general ailment.	Look for other symptoms before commencing treatment.
Blindness with abnormalities in the lens of the eye.	Cataracts.	Surgery is possible, but rarely practical.
Blindness, no obvious lesions in the eye.	Possible Cerebrocorical Necrosis. Due to thiamine deficiency Encephalitis ie. brain infection or Listeriosis.	Thiamine injections are usually beneficial. Antibiotic injections may be helpful. Need to use those that pass the blood brain barrier eg. ampicillin.
Yellow colour in the white of the eye.	Jaundice - usually the result of copper poisoning. This may be due to excess copper in the food, but may be over medication ie. misuse of copper injection.	Oral dose of sodium sulphate may help, but generally poor prognosis.
Membranes of the eye pale or white.	Anaemia due to worms or fluke or deficiency of iron in the diet.	Treat with anthelmintic if indicated. Iron by injection. Vitamin B12 also useful.
Membranes of the eye dark and congested.	Circulatory difficulties as part of more generalised disease eg. Pneumonia or Toxaemias.	Check for other symptoms. If in doubt see vet.
Eyes sunk into sockets.	Dehydration usually as the result of scouring.	Electrolytes and fluid therapy and treat cause of dehydration.
EARS		
One or both ears swollen.	Abscess or blood blister ie. haematoma.	Drain abscess and inject antibiotic. Haematoma, leave to absorb naturally, but this will result in 'cauliflower ear.'
One ear drooping with possible discharge from ear canal.	No specific bacterial infection or may be Listeriosis.	Antibiotic. If Listeriosis then consider source of infection eg. silage pit. Also practise good hygiene to limit the spread of infection.
SKIN AND COAT		
Loss of hair with itch and some skin thickening.	Mange due to Sarcoptes scabiei or Chorioptic mange if lesions are confined to the legs or heels. Skin scrapings required for diagnosis.	Pour on Ivermectin preparation.
Itchy places around the head, ears and legs.	Sheep scab due to Psoroptic mite infestation.	Gamma benzene hexachloride. Ivermectin orally or pour on Ivermectin.
Severe itching with nervous signs.	Scrapie due to infection by small virus-like particles (NB. notifiable disease).	No treatment. All infected animals should be slaughtered.

Signs of Disease	Causes	Treatment and Prevention
SKIN AND COAT CONTINUED		
Small nodules or spots over the chest and shoulders, some irritation.	Demodectic mange infection. Skin scraping required for diagnosis.	Treatment difficult. Try Malathion or Rotenone compounds.
Loss of hair in small patches anywhere on the body. Not itchy.	Ringworm usually due to Trichophyton infection (NB. infectious to people).	Topical antifungal agents.
Multiple skin eruptions and swellings.	Possible allergic reaction due to inhaled, ingested or contact allergen.	Antihistamine or corticosteroid injections. May need to change feed.
Swellings/abscesses around the rear or hind end.	Caseous lymphadenitis due to a type of tuberculosis (NB. notifiable disease). Rare in the UK.	No treatment effective.
BREATHING		
Rapid breathing.	Stress due to pain or overheating or exercise.	Remove the source of the stress and the symptoms should resolve quite quickly.
	Pneumonia commonly due to bacterial infection eg Pasteurellosis.	Injection of antibiotic required. Reduce stress, if indoors. Vaccine available for Pasteurella infection.
	Parasitic Pneumonia due to lungworm infection.	Anthelmintic eg. Ivermectin or Levamisole required or Fenbendazole.
	Bluetongue (NB. notifiable disease).	No effective treatment for Bluetongue - vaccinate and control midges.
Slow progressive onset of rapid breathing.	Rare form of C.A.E. ie. Caprine Arthritis and Encephalitis.	No treatment. Slaughter all affected animals.
Shallow breathing.	Asleep or in terminal stage of illness.	If unable to wake the animal get the vet ASAP.
Coughing.	Respiratory infection eg. Pneumonia. Due to infection by bacteria, virus or parasite (see above).	Antibiotic, anti-inflammatory and mucolytic drugs. Anthelmintic for lungworm. Get vet to check diagnosis.
	Inhalation Pneumonia following faulty drenching or dosing.	Antibiotic to control secondary infection. Improve drenching technique.
TEMPERATURE (normal range is 101.5 to 102.5°F)		
Raised.	Usually means an infection, but may be the result of heat, stress or pain. Check again. May be incorrect reading.	Check for other symptoms. If in doubt check with a vet. Antibiotic for infection.
Lowered.	If correct may be terminally ill.	Check for other symptoms eg. diarrhoea. Give symptomatic treatment until diagnosis is made and warm patient up gradually.

Signs of Disease	Causes	Treatment and Prevention
DUNG		
Constipation.	May be the result of Acetonaemia ie. negative energy balance in first month after kidding. Could also be the sequel to digestive disorders or a fever.	Intravenous glucose and corticosteroids, propylene glycol or glycerine by mouth. Laxative ie. liquid paraffin or epsom salts in a bran mash.
Scouring. No blood in diarrhoea.	Parasitic gastroenteritis ie. worms. Many species may be involved. Faecal sample required to make diagnosis. Chronic Fasciolisis ie. chronic fluke infection.	Dose with anthelmintic and move onto clean pasture. Dose with anthelmintic for fluke infection. See vet if in doubt. Drain land and get rid of snail which is the intermediate host.
Scouring, light in colour.	Ruminal acidosis due to animal eating too many concentrates or cereal.	Remove concentrate diet. Give carbohydrate by mouth. Multivitamins and antihistamines may help.
Scouring after change of diet or moving onto new pasture.	Similar to above. Nutritional upset due to change of diet or lush pasture.	Increase roughage in diet eg. hay and symptoms should disappear. Change diet slowly.
Dung persistently soft and loose. Animal very thin.	Johne's Disease (NB. notifiable in N. Ireland) due to infection by Mycobacterium Johnei.	No treatment. Euthanase on welfare grounds.
Scour with occasional blood seen.	Possible Salmonella infection (NB. infectious to people).	Antibiotic and fluid therapy. Careful nursing required. Very guarded outlook.
Scouring with blood and mucus seen. Animal very depressed.	Enterotoxaemia due to clostridial infection.	Antibiotic in high doses and anti-inflammatory injections plus fluid therapy. Vaccine useful to control disease.
Scouring, loss of colour in coat, anaemia.	Consider copper or cobalt deficiency. Need blood test for diagnosis.	Give copper or cobalt by injection or orally, but only after diagnosis has been reached.
BLOAT		
Abdominal distention of left side of abdomen.	Gas not being belched from rumen. Could be due to obstruction ie. foreign body (unlikely in a goat) or failure in the mechanism to allow belching. Frothy bloat (most likely type in adults) where gas and stomach contents are mixed as a froth. Usually caused by overeating, especially on a lush diet.	If bloat due to obstruction, remove it or push it into the rumen. If this is not possible the vet will insert trocar and cannula to relieve abdominal distention. If a frothy bloat use stomach drench of silicone or vegetable oil preparations. Remove from suspect pasture or restrict access. Feed hay prior to turning out.
Bloat with distention on both sides of the abdomen.	Severe bloat. Animal will be close to death.	May require emergency trocarisation. Get the vet.

Signs of Disease	Causes	Treatment and Prevention
BLOAT CONTINUED		
Abdominal distention with mammary enlargement.	Pregnant, or if has not been with male, false pregnancy.	If not pregnant, prostaglandins or corticosteroids will cause a 'cloud burst' and the animal will return to normal.
URINE		
Diffuse swelling along belly from navel backwards with or without urine dribbling from sheath.	Urolithiasis due to calculi blocking urethra. Particularly common in male castrates.	Relaxant drugs if partial blockage. Surgery or euthanasia for severe cases. Check diet. Salt in diet may prevent new cases.
Discoloured urine, often dark red in colour.	Clostridial infection. Rare in goats.	Antibiotic and fluid therapy. Poor prognosis. Vaccine as prevention.
Blood in urine.	Bacterial infection or Urolithiasis or both.	Antibiotic (plus see above).
Pain in abdomen; seen as getting up and lying down frequently, teeth grinding and kicking at belly.	Colic due to bloat, or Urolithiasis or intestinal blockage.	Muscle relaxants or pain killers. Surgery if indicated will lead to poor prognosis.
LAMENESS		
Feet.	Bacterial infection in the foot eg. foot rot or foot abscess or foot scald. Commonly due to Fusiformis species or, if abscess, Corynebacteria.	Pare foot where appropriate and dress with topical spray. Inject antibiotic when required. Keep feet dry and clean and use foot baths with formalin as prevention.
Blisters around the coronet. Swelling around and above hoof.	Foot and Mouth Disease (NB. notifiable disease). Bluetongue (NB. notifiable disease).	Check for ulcers in mouth. If in any doubt call the vet. No treatment. Vaccinate and control midges.
Limbs.	Injury eg. fracture, nerve damage, puncture wounds or strain. Clostridial infection eg. Blackleg. Animal will be actutely ill.	All but the most minor may need vet attention. Treat as required by symptoms. Large doses of antibiotic and antisera. Vaccinate to prevent.
Swollen joints.	Caprine Arthritis and Encephalomyelitis (C.A.E.). Erysipelas or other joint infections.	None. Euthanasia often required on welfare grounds. Keep away from all young animals. Antibiotic and good hygiene required. Clean pens and dips.
Reluctant to move on front feet, taking weight on hind.	Laminitis ie. inflammation in the lamina of the foot, due to bacterial toxins in blood stream or may be just overweight or animal may have gorged on too rich a diet.	Pain killers and anti-inflammatory drugs. Bathe feet in warm water. Check diet.
Painful joints and stiff with tendency for bones to fracture easily.	Osteomalacia due to dietary imbalance of calcium, phosphorus and vitamin D. Often the result of pregnancy and lactation.	Oral and injectable calcium and vitamin D preparations. Check and maintain adequate diet.

Signs of Disease	Causes	Treatment and Prevention
INFERTILITY - FEMALE		
Failure to come into season.	Pregnant. May be false pregnancy due to hormone imbalance.	Vet may be required to check for pregnancy.
	Low body weight or deficiency disease eg. manganese or copper or vitamin E /selenium.	Check diagnosis with blood samples before undertaking any treatment.
	Ovarian problems which in the young goat may be congenital.	If treating individual it may be worth trying treatment but if congenital, cull from herd. See vet.
Comes into season but does not conceive.	Possible genital tract infection.	Antibiotic or cull from herd.
	Hormone imbalance.	May be treatable on individual basis by vet.
Abortion.	Infection most likely cause eg. Toxoplasma, Brucellosis (NB. infectious to people), Campylobacter, Listeriosis, tick borne fever, Salmonella and fungal infections.	All abortions should be investigated properly. Treat all as potentially hazardous to people. Good hygiene is essential at all times. Isolate affected animals until a diagnosis is made.
	Isolated cases may be due to poor handling and clumsy management.	Check and improve on management.
Vaginal discharge - clear with or without blood staining.	If pregnant, may be about to give birth or abort. Slight discharge may be apparent when in season.	Get experienced help to check.
Purulent smelly discharge with or without afterbirth being retained.	If not pregnant, primary infection of genital tract. If after giving birth, Metritis due to infection with or without retention of afterbirth. Dead kids may still be retained in uterus.	Antibiotic by injection and in uterine pessaries or uterine irrigation. Remove retained afterbirth if possible and any retained, dead kids.
INFERTILITY - MALE		
	Specific infection of the testicle(s).	Better to cull animal than to attempt treatment.
	Deficiency disease eg. vitamin A or zinc.	Vitamin or zinc supplements.
	Lameness eg. sore back legs or feet making it difficult or painful for the animal to mount.	Should be self evident on careful observation. Get vet to check and treat any lameness.
	Sores around sheath or scrotum may inhibit mating - check for Orf.	Localised treatment with antibiotic may help.
MASTITIS		
Milk very thick after kidding.	Normal colostrum.	Milk will clear after a few days.
Clots in milk.	Mild form of Mastitis. Many bacteria might be involved, but probably a Streptococcus.	Intra-mammary antibiotic required.

Signs of Disease	Causes	Treatment and Prevention
MASTITIS CONTINUED		
Milk very watery and udder often very sore and red.	Acute Mastitis due to E. coli or Pasteurella or Staphylococcus aureus.	Antibiotic, both intra-mammary and injectable.
Udder cold, goat very ill, blood stained fluid present at teat.	Peracute Mastitis with gangrene, usually due to Staph. aureus or Pasteurella infection.	May be necessary to amputate teat to allow drainage. Antibiotic, anti-inflammatory drugs and electrolytes may be required. Very grave prognosis.
Udder normal temperature but hard, no milk can be expressed.	Chronic Mastitis. Blocked teat canal.	Probably no effective treatment, but try antibiotic injection. Get vet to check and unblock if possible.
Red sores over the udder area.	Orf ie. virus infection.	Antibiotic will help stop spread of infection.
Milk taint. Goats' milk should taste similar to cows' milk.	Source of taint could be food eg. silage, turnips etc. Acetonaemia. Presence of male goats, poor hygiene when milking. Some medications.	Check diet. Fluids, steroids, propylene glycol. Get vet to check when source is not apparent.
BEHAVIOUR		
Loss of appetite.	Any infection causing a rise in temperature. Pain - check mouth for sores. Check for abdominal pain eg. teeth grinding and grunting.	Check for the symptoms before starting treatment. Treatment depends on cause of pain and definite diagnosis required - see vet.
Slow progressive loss of appetite in pregnant animal and finally recumbency.	Pregnancy Toxaemia due to energy deficiency caused by faulty feeding procedure. Less common than in sheep.	Glycerol, propylene glycol, steroids and anabolic steroid. Abortion may be necessary. Ensure adequate diet and exercise in last half of pregnancy.
Slow progressive loss of appetite in lactating animal.	Acetonaemia due to negative energy balance as result of faulty feeding.	Treatment similar to that for Pregnancy Toxaemia.
Fairly sudden loss of appetite and then recumbency in later pregnancy and after kidding.	Hypocalcaemia due to lack of calcium in circulation.	Give calcium intravenously or under the skin.
Recumbency with fits and foaming at the mouth.	Hypomagnesaemia due to low levels of magnesium in the blood stream. More common on lush pasture after kidding.	Magnesium injection given under the skin. Feed magnesium rich food. Restrict time on lush pasture. Magnesium boluses.
Walking in circles and head pressing.	Middle ear infection or Listeriosis. Gid (Sturdy) ie. tapeworm cyst in brain.	Antibiotic. Avoid silage feeding. Good hygiene essential at kidding time as Listerella can cause abortions. Surgery to remove cyst. Routine tapeworm dosing of all dogs.

Signs of Disease	Causes	Treatment and Prevention
BEHAVIOUR CONTINUED		
Head pressing with peculiar high stepping gait, then recumbency.	Louping Ill due to virus infection.	Antisera may be useful if used early. Vaccine available. Control the tick which is the intermediate host.
Progressive lameness with swollen joints and eventual paralysis.	Caprine Arthritis and Encephalitis (C.A.E.) due to virus infection.	No treatment. Isolate all infected animals. Blood test available.
Intense itch with loss of condition despite good appetite, recumbency, head raised with lip nibbling.	Scrapie due to infection by small virus like particles (NB. notifiable disease).	Slaughter all affected animals.
General stiffness, anxious and often immoble.	Tetanus due to infection by Clostridium tetani in the wound.	Antisera antibiotic sedation. Vaccine available.
SUDDEN DEATH		
Without prior warning.	Anthrax ie. infection with Bacillus anthracis (NB. notifiable disease and infectious to people). Any of the clostridial diseases eg. Enterotoxaemia. Plant poisoning eg. yew or laurel. Lightning strike or electocution.	Rare. Source of infection usually contaminated feed. Vaccines are available and effective. Goats are very inquisitive. Never leave hedge or tree clipping where animals can reach them. Post-mortem should be able to show scorch marks on the skin. Get qualified person to check electrical wiring etc.

DIAGNOSTIC GUIDE TO KID AILMENTS AND TREATMENT

Signs of Disease	Causes	Treatment and Prevention
HEAD AND FACE		
Nasal Discharge.	Pneumonia due to virus or bacterial infection. Most common infection is due to Pasteurella species. Bacterial or fungal infection in upper respiratory tract.	Antibiotic for most cases. If animal is kept indoors check ventilation. Vaccine available for Pasteurella control. Antibiotic or antifungal preparations after swabbing to make diagnosis.
Ulcers on lips, tongue and dental pad.	Foot and Mouth disease (NB. notifiable disease).	Check for other symptoms eg. blisters around feet. if suspicious inform vet.
Scabs on lips, nostrils and eye lids.	Orf ie. infection by Paravaccinia virus.	Topical ointments and sprays can stop secondary bacterial infection. Isolate affected animals. Vaccine available.
Scabs on face ie. around eyes, ears and base of horns.	Facial eczema due to bacterial infection ie. Staphylococcus aureus. Not common but may be complicated by fly worry.	Antibiotic and check to make sure trough space is adequate. Insecticides can be used and head protected by head cap.
Loss of hair on face, especially around the eyes.	Ringworm, usually due to Trichophyton verrucosum. Rare condition but more common than in sheep (NB. infectious to people).	Topical antifungal agents.
Salivation and drooling from the mouth.	Viral infection eg. Orf or Foot and Mouth disease (see above). Actinobacillosis ie. bacterial infection in the mouth and jaw bone and elsewhere. Uncommon in young animals. Consider possibility of foreign body stuck in mouth eg. thorn or bramble.	See above. Antibiotic or sodium iodide intravenous weekly or potassium iodide orally daily. Have a good look with torch and mouth gag.
Swollen lip and blue tongue.	Bluetongue (NB. notifiable disease).	No effective treatment. Vaccinate and control midges.
EYES		
Watery discharge from one or both eyes.	Entropion ie. inturned eye lid.	Minor surgery required.
White discharge from one or both eyes, sometimes with damage to the surface of the eye.	Infectious Kerato-conjunctivitis due to infection by Rickettsia or Chlamydia bacteria.	Subconjunctival injection (job for the vet) or topical antibiotic ointment. Control is difficult. Reduce crowding. Control flies.
Discharge from one eye with or without eye damage.	Look for foreign body in the eye eg. hay seed.	Careful search required and then remove. Antibiotic ointment after removal.
Swollen eye lids.	Allergic reaction.	Antihistamine or corticosteroid injections. May have to move pastures.

Signs of Disease	Causes	Treatment and Prevention
EYES CONTINUED		
Eyes dull and lifeless.	Animal may be in pain or suffering from any general ailment.	Look for other symptoms before commencing treatment.
Blindness with abnormalities in the lens of the eye.	Cataracts.	Surgery is possible but rarely practical.
Blindness with no obvious lesions in the eye.	Possible Cerebrocortical Necrosis. Due to thiamine deficiency. Encephalitis ie. brain infection or Listeriosis.	Thiamine injections are usually beneficial. Antibiotic injections may be helpful. Need to use those that pass the blood brain barrier eg. ampicillin.
Yellow colour in the white of the eye.	Jaundice - usually the result of copper poisoning. This may be due to excess copper in the food, but may be over medication ie. misuse of copper injection.	Oral dose of sodium sulphate may help, but generally poor prognosis.
Membranes of the eye pale or white.	Anaemia due to worms or fluke or deficiency of iron in the diet.	Treat with anthelmintic if indicated. Iron by injection. Vitamin B12 also useful.
Membranes of the eye dark and congested.	Circulatory difficulties as part of more generalised disease eg. Pneumonia or Toxaemias.	Check for other symptoms. If in doubt see vet.
Eyes sunk into sockets.	Dehydration usually as the result of scouring.	Electrolytes and fluid therapy and treat the cause of dehydration.
EARS		
One or both ears swollen.	Abscess or blood blister ie. haematoma.	Drain abscess and inject antibiotic. Haematoma, leave to absorb naturally, but this will result in 'cauliflower ear.'
One ear drooping with possible discharge from ear canal.	No specific bacterial infection or may be Listeriosis.	Antibiotic. if Listeriosis then consider source of infection eg. silage pit. Also practise good hygiene to limit spread of infection.
SKIN AND COAT		
Loss of hair with itch and some skin thickening.	Mange due to Sarcoptes scabiei or Chorioptic mange if lesions are confined to the legs or heels. Skin scrapings required for diagnosis.	Repeat washings with organo-phosphorus compounds or similar recommended products.
Itchy places around the head, ears and legs.	Sheep scab due to Psoroptic mite infestation.	Use sheep scab dip preparations containing Diazinon or Propetamphos.
Loss of coat with severe itiching. Parasites found.	Lice infestation.	Dip or spray or dust with recommended products eg. organo-phosphorus compounds or Gamma benzene hexachloride. Ivermectin orally.

Signs of Disease	Causes	Treatment and Prevention
SKIN AND COAT CONTINUED		
Severe itching with nervous signs.	Scrapie due to infection by small virus - like particle (NB. notifiable disease).	No treatment. All infected animals should be slaughtered.
Small nodules or spots over the chest and shoulders, some irritation.	Demodectic mange infection. Skin scraping required for diagnosis.	Treatment difficult. Try Malathion or Rotenone compounds.
Loss of hair in small patches anywhere on body. Not itchy.	Ringworm usually due to Trichophyton infection (NB. infectious to people).	Topical antifungal agents.
Multiple skin eruptions and swellings.	Possible allergic reaction due to inhaled, ingested or contact allergen.	Antihistamine or corticosteroid injections. May need to change feed.
BREATHING		
Rapid breathing.	Pneumonia usually due to bacterial infection eg. Pasteurellosis.	Antibiotic. Reduce stress, check ventilation. Vaccine available.
	Stress due to pain, overheating or exercise.	Remove the source of the stress and the symptoms should resolve quickly.
Shallow breathing.	Asleep or in terminal stage of illness.	If unable to wake get the vet ASAP.
Coughing.	Respiratory disease eg. Pneumonia.	Antibiotic, anti-inflammatory drugs and mucolytics.
	Inhalation Pneumonia following faulty drenching and dosing.	Antibiotic to control secondary infection. Improve dosing technique.
TEMPERATURE (normal range is 101.5 - 102.5°F)		
Raised.	Usually means an infection has set in, but could be due to pain, stress or weather conditions.	Check for other symptoms. If in doubt check with vet. Antibiotic for infection.
Lowered.	Check again. May be incorrect reading or technique. Hypothermia can be a killer in young kids. Animal may be terminally ill.	Raise body temperature with heat lamps or equivalent. Check for other symptoms eg. diarrhoea.
Shivering.	May be early stages of hypothermia.	See above. Check for draughts if indoors. If outdoors, is there adequate shelter? Has the youngster fed recently?
DUNG		
Constipation.	Uncommon but can be one of the symptoms of wet mouth.	Check for other symptoms. Liquid paraffin useful 1 -2 teaspoonfuls.
Scouring. Young kids, no blood in diarrhoea.	Bacterial (eg. E. coli) or viral infection (eg. Rotavirus).	Antibiotic and electrolytes. Keep the patient warm. Colostrum essential for prevention as is good hygiene.
Scouring with blood in diarrhoea, animal very ill.	Enterotoxaemia due to clostridial infection.	Antibiotic and anti-inflammatory injections plus electrolytes. Keep the patient warm. Vaccine useful to control disease.

Signs of Disease	Causes	Treatment and Prevention
DUNG CONTINUED		
Kid at least 3-4 weeks old with diarrhoea, some blood may be present.	Coccidiosis, usually infection with Eimeria species.	Oral antibacterials eg. Amprolium of sulphadimidine. Avoid overcrowding and wet areas. Prophylactic medication in the feed may be used.
Older kids with diarrhoea, no blood.	Parasitic gastroenteritis ie. worms. These include Haemonchus, Ostertagia, Trichostrongylus, Nematodirus and Oesophagostomum species.	Anthelmintic to all affected animals. Put onto worm free pasture after worming the kids.
Diarrhoea with no signs of infection.	Nutritional scour due to lush pasture or sudden increase in feed.	Remove from diet and put onto hay and water diet until recovered.
BLOAT		
Abdominal distention of left side of abdomen.	Gas not being belched from rumen or abomasum (true stomach). Could be due to obstruction in gullet or failure of the belching mechanism, or frothy bloat where gas and fluid are mixed as a froth.	Dose with silicone or oil preparations. Pass stomach tube if necessary. Get vet to check diet. If bloat due to lush diet of lucerne or clover, remove from pasture and feed hay and water when distention is relieved.
Bloat with distention on both sides of abdomen.	Uncommon in young kids, except those bottle fed. Severe bloat. Animal will be close to death.	Emergency. May require trocarisation. Get vet.
Swelling under belly at navel.	Navel infection. Umbilical hernia.	Antibiotic. Dip navel at birth with iodine or spray with antibiotic. If small, no action required. If large, surgery may be required.
URINE		
Diffuse swelling under navel in older kids.	Urolithiasis due to calculi blocking urethra.	Relaxant drugs if partial blockage. Surgery or euthanasia for severe cases. Check diet. Salt in diet may prevent new cases.
Discoloured urine, often dark red colour.	Clostridial infection. Rare in kids.	Antibiotic and fluid therapy. Poor prognosis. Vaccine to prevent.
Pain in abdomen; seen as lying down and getting up frequently, teeth grinding and kicking.	Colic due to bloat, Urolithiasis or intestinal blockage.	Muscle relaxants, pain killers. Surgery if indicated will give a poor prognosis.
LAMENESS		
Feet.	Bacterial infection in the foot eg. foot rot, foot abscess or foot scald. Commonly due to Fusiformis species or, if abscess, Corynebacteria. Virus infection eg. Foot and Mouth disease (NB. notifiable disease).	Pare foot where appropriate and dress with topical spray. Inject antibiotic. Keep feet dry and clean and use foot baths with 5% formalin as prevention. Check for ulcers in mouth. If in doubt call the vet.

Signs of Disease	Causes	Treatment and Prevention
LAMENESS CONTINUED		
Limbs.	Injury eg. fracture, nerve damage, puncture wounds or strain.	All but the most minor may need vet attention. Treat as required by symptoms.
	Clostridial infection eg Blackleg. Rare in young goats.	Large doses of antibiotic and antisera. Vaccinate to prevent.
Swollen joints.	Joint Ill ie. bacterial infection in the joint(s) eg. Erysipelas or C. pyogenes.	Antibiotic and good hygiene required. Clean pens and foot dips. Dip navels at birth in iodine or spray with antibiotic.
Deformed limbs.	Rickets due to imbalance of calcium, phosphorus and vitamin D.	Oral and injectable calcium and vitamin D preparations. Check and maintain adequate diet.
Softening of jaw bones and frequent fractures.	Excess phosphorus in the diet.	Give extra calcium and ensure a balanced diet.
Stiff limbs and sometimes difficulty in standing.	Vitamin E/selenium deficiency.	Vitamin E and selenium injections. Nutritional supplements.
BEHAVIOUR		
Loss of appetite.	Any infection causing a rise in temperature.	Check for other symptoms before starting any treatment.
	Pain. Check mouth for sores, check for abdominal pain.	Treatment depends on cause of pain. Pain killers, anti-inflammatory drugs and antibiotic may all be helpful.
	Pain causing lameness is unlikely to cause loss of appetite.	
Kids born weak with tremors and hair abnormalities.	Border disease due to viral infection.	No treatment. Isolate all infected animals and their mothers who will be carrying the infection.
Progressive hind leg paralysis with lameness and swollen joints in older kids.	C.A.E. due to viral infection.	No treatment. Isolate all infected animals.
Born dead or weak with uncoordinated leg movements and swaying.	Swayback. Due to copper deficiency in the mother.	Very little can be done for clinical cases. Prevent by giving mother copper injections or boluses or oral copper supplements.
Blindness and walking in circles in older kids.	Cerebrocortical necrosis due to thiamine deficiency.	High levels of thiamine by injection.
Walking in circles and head pressing.	Middle ear infection or Listeriosis.	Antibiotic. Avoid silage. Good hygiene essential at kidding time.
Head pressing with peculiar gait, then recumbency.	Louping Ill due to virus infection.	Antisera may be useful if used early. Vaccine available. Control ticks which are the intermediate host.

Signs of Disease	Causes	Treatment and Prevention
BEHAVIOUR CONTINUED		
Kids dull and weak usually within a few hours or days of birth.	Hypothermia as the result of bad weather or inadequate feeding.	Rewarm gently. Feed by stomach tube if cannot suckle. Provide adequate shelter and make sure the youngster has had an adequate colostrum intake.
SUDDEN DEATH		
Without prior warning.	Anthrax ie. infection with Bacillus anthracis (NB. notifiable disease and infectious to people)..	Rare. Source of infection is usually contaminated feed.
	Any of the clostridial diseases eg. Enterotoxaemia.	Vaccines are available and effective.
	Plant poisoning eg. yew or laurel.	Kids are inquisitive. Never leave hedge or tree clippings around.
	Lightning strike or electrocution.	Post-mortem should be able to show scorch marks on the skin. Get a qualified person to check all electrical wiring etc.

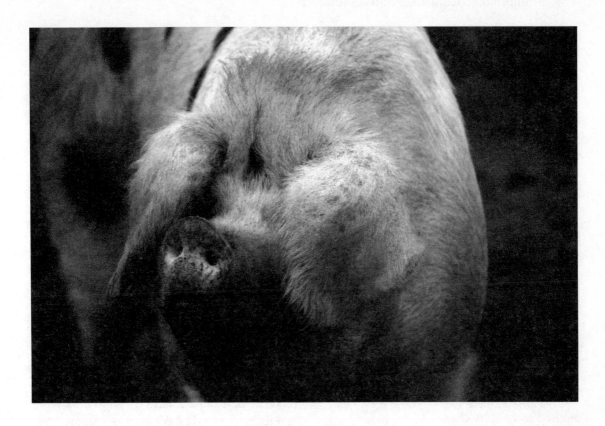

Chapter Five

PIG AILMENTS

By Carol Harris

The rare breeds of pig tend to be quite hardy and healthy on the whole and traditionally kept pigs of whatever breed are likely to be healthier than intensively reared animals because they have freedom of movement, exposure to fresh air and sunlight, access to grass and naturally occurring minerals in the soil and better mental health arising from social activity.

There are, however, various things it is important to know about pig health and this chapter addresses the major topics. If in doubt you should always consult your vet or a more experienced pig keeper but, as you become more familiar with pigs in general, and your own animals in particular, you will learn to recognise signs of good health and poor health and be able to act accordingly.

A healthy pig is physically and mentally active. It looks alert and lively, responds to people and other animals, has a good appetite, has a shiny coat and clear eyes, passes well-formed stools and exhibits behaviour that is consistent with its age, temperament and training.

A pig that is not healthy can exhibit various signs – and some of the most common (although not all appearing at the same time) are:

• Poor appetite and thirst – or overeating and drinking
• Listlessness – and sometimes an unwillingness to get up at all
• Uncharacteristic behaviour (anxiety, aggression and so forth)
• A dull coat
• Watery eyes
• Lameness or stiffness
• Constant scratching or rubbing against objects
• Hair loss
• Standing hunched up
• Rapid breathing or coughing
• Discharge from nose, mouth, eyes or vagina
• Unusually coloured urine or excessive or limited urine production
• Unusual colour, consistency and volume of dung
• Vomiting
• Wounds or bleeding
• Abnormal swellings
• Abnormal temperature – either very high or very low

Most animal keepers will be able to tell if their own animals are unwell as they will somehow just seem slightly different from usual. Major health issues will be easy to spot but minor ones may sometimes be overlooked as their symptoms are so slight. Daily checks on all your animals are important so you can spot any symptoms early and take appropriate action.

There are some routine things you should do to maintain your pigs' health such as worming or vaccination, although if are organic these may not be permissible as routine operations.

Worms

Roundworms can affect pigs. These include lungworms, threadworms, nodular worms and kidney worms. The commonest form of worms are Ascarids, which normally live in the small intestine. These are white worms, about 30cm (12in) long and about ½cm (¼in) thick. Adult female worms produce up to two hundred thousand eggs a day, which are passed out in the faeces and, in optimum weather conditions, can develop to infectious stage in three weeks. Otherwise development of the eggs may be prolonged over several months. The eggs are very resistant to freezing and drying, although exposure to sunlight will kill them in a few weeks. Pigs become infected by eating the eggs along with food or water, or in the case of young pigs, during suckling. The eggs hatch in the intestine and the larvae penetrate the intestine wall and get into the blood stream and are carried first to the liver and then, five to six days later, the lungs. A cough is the prominent symptom of worm infection and Ascarid pneumonia in young pigs can cause death. Animals that survive lung infestation may be permanently stunted.

The worms can also migrate to other parts of the body, including the placenta. Once in the lungs, the larvae travel up to the throat and are swallowed and pass into the small intestine where they reach maturity in eight to nine weeks and are finally expelled. The adult worms cause little damage to the pig, although they can cause some digestive problems – they can also burrow into ulcers or abrasions and can penetrate the intestines, causing peritonitis. If lots of larvae are acquired at one time, they can cause damage by mass migration through the lungs and also damage the liver, where white spots can be seen. The first sign of infestation in young pigs is a soft, moist cough, which can be transitory. Symptoms may be lack of appetite and failure to put on weight or loss of existing weight. The presence of runts in litters can also be indicative of worms.

Lungworms are slender, white worms about 5cm (2in) long. They are found in the lungs, where eggs are laid that are carried up into the throat and swallowed. They turn into embryos that are ready to hatch and are passed out in the faeces. They are then eaten by earthworms and begin their development. Each earthworm can harbour up to two thousand larvae and, when earthworms are eaten by pigs, the larvae are freed in the intestine, go through the intestinal wall, get into the lymph system and are carried to the heart and then the lungs. They develop further in the lungs. Lungworm eggs can remain viable in the soil for several years. The main symptoms are a husky cough and diarrhoea as well as poor growth and loss of condition. High levels of infestation can cause pneumonia and death. Young pigs are the most susceptible – resistance tends to develop at about six months of age. Lowered bodily resistance is a predisposing factor, so a good diet is essential. Pigs kept on land that has had pigs grazing on it for a long time are more likely to get these worms because of high levels of infestation in the soil, so clean land, available through crop rotation, is much better if available. Reducing the earthworm population by periodically keeping ducks on the land can help, although earthworms of course do the soil a lot of good generally, so this may not be a desired course of action.

Regular worming will prevent your pigs from becoming infested and can also save you money on food, although, if you farm organically, you will probably not be allowed to worm routinely as one of the principles of organic farming is maintenance of land that is worm-free. Worming is carried out either by oral application of a liquid worming product such as Panacur or by injection of a multi-pur-

pose anti-parasite product such as Dectomax or Ivomec. Pigs should be wormed at about eight weeks of age and then at least twice a year. (You should also worm females when they are put with a boar and again seven to ten days before farrowing to avoid the piglets being born with worms, which can be potentially fatal).

External Parasites

Lice

Lice are one of the most common of all parasites. They live on the pig and, when they lay their eggs, they are glued to the pig's hairs, close to the skin, especially on the lower half of the abdomen, the neck and jowl, the ears, the shoulders, the insides of the legs and the flanks. The lice can lay three to four eggs a day, which hatch in twelve to twenty days and grow very quickly, becoming mature in about twelve days. If they fall off the pig through scratching or other means they can only survive for two or three days, so pig houses are unlikely to remain infected if there are no pigs in them for a few days. Lice irritate the pigs' skin considerably and can also be a transmitting agent for the pig pox virus. Pigs with lice may fail to feed properly and can be more susceptible to other diseases and parasites. Treatment of lice is simple, with either a topical powder, a poured-on liquid or a multipurpose anti-parasite injection. Commercial louse powders are easily available and simply require the pigs to be dusted with the product every few weeks.

Mange

Mange is a skin disease caused by mites. There are two species of these mites:

Sarcoptic Mange

Sarcoptic Mange is more common and involves a burrowing mite. The infestation usually begins on the head – usually round the eyes, nose or ears (it is often inside the ear which can become filled with a dry, crusty scurf); it then spreads over the neck and shoulders, along the back and sides and finally the whole body. With Sarcoptic Mange the animal scratches and liberates tissue fluids that coagulate, dry and form crusts on the skin. The skin becomes inflamed and swollen, it thickens and wrinkles and frequent rubbing may give it a leathery appearance and much of the pig's hair is either rubbed off or falls off, giving a dry, scurfy appearance. Constant rubbing can result in raw areas that become scabby and crack – there can then be blood and serum exuded, together with a bad smell. The pigs often shake their heads a lot and rub them against surfaces. If untreated the animals become emaciated and may die – often from exhaustion. As the parasites only survive for just over two weeks away from the host, leaving the pig houses empty for a while can avoid infection of other animals.

Demodectic Mange

This is caused by microscopic mites that inhabit the hair follicles or sebaceous glands. It has little effect in healthy animals but ones in poor states of nutrition can have high levels of infestation, which cause skin lesions. The lesions usually appear first on the snout or around the eyes and spread slowly from there to the underside of the neck, the stomach and the inner sides of the hind legs and other areas with thin, tender skin. The skin becomes red and is scurfy, scaly and hard. Red nodules may appear which can rupture and leave cavities that discharge pus in which the mites live.

With both kinds of mange the animal is likely to be seen shaking its head due to the irritation caused by the condition. Treatment involves spraying or injecting or both. However, animals that are very badly affected with Demodectic Mange do not always respond well to treatment.

Sometimes pigs can lose their coats without parasites being present. Kune Kunes, for example, often seem to lose patches of coat for no apparent reason. The coat always grows back in time but does look very unsightly for a period. If your animals do lose their coat, you should check their diet to make sure they have adequate nutrition and make sure they don't have parasites; if there is no obvious sign then simply wait for it to re-grow, or treat the skin with oil or a natural health product to aid re-growth.

Diarrhoea

Diarrhoea in pigs is called scouring. It can occur for a number of reasons and, if very temporary, is not a serious issue. If it is prolonged, however, it can cause dehydration (sometimes fatal) and is generally a symptom of an underlying ailment that needs dealing with. Both adult pigs and piglets can suffer from scouring. In piglets it may be due to the quality of the sow's milk, a lack of colostrum (the initial milk from the sow that helps give immunity from diseases), anaemia, the change to solid food and so forth. In adults it can arise from infectious gastroenteritis, sudden changes of food, too high protein levels in food, too much food or excessive amounts of certain fresh foods (such as soft fruit or fodder beet), worms and other causes. To protect new born piglets against enteritis you can vaccinate your females six and two weeks before they produce their litters. If you have pigs that are scouring you can use a powder in the drinking water (Tylan is the most common), although it is difficult to use in automatic drinkers as you don't know how much is being taken by individual pigs Alternatively, you can treat with clay/kaolin-based products, use a natural remedy or take advice from your vet about other prescription drugs. Diarrhoea should always be diagnosed before antibiotic treatment is applied.

Colds

Pigs can get colds and exhibit similar symptoms to people if they do so – a runny nose being the commonest sign. There is little to be done in these cases apart from ensuring the pig is kept warm and fed well, however, pneumonia can result in extreme cases and can be lethal.

Pneumonia

This may be a more serious problem when air space in pig houses is very humid, so good ventilation is important; however, an extremely dry atmosphere is not recommended either. With viral pneumonia the infection can be quite dramatic if introduced into a herd that has had no previous exposure to it, and mortality may be high. In fact few herds have had no contact with the disease so most cases of pneumonia are of the chronic, rather than acute, variety. The symptoms include a transient diarrhoea, followed by a dry cough. The breathing rate is fast and some animals show acute respiratory distress and a high temperature. The cough may disappear or persist almost indefinitely. The coat may also lack shine and the skin may have a grey tinge. Affected pigs can fail to thrive. Pigs may be carriers of viral pneumonia, although they show no clinical signs. Once the disease is established in a herd it tends to remain indefinitely in an endemic form. Warm, dry, draught-proof houses and good feed reduce the effects of this ailment. The disease spreads through droplet infection through the air, so uninfected clean pigs must be separated in the open by at least six feet from possibly infected pigs and never put in the same building. Treatment is by antibiotics.

Infectious Atrophic Rhinitis

This is a stress-related disease, often referred to as 'snuffles' that is caused by a bacterium and precipitated by such things as very early weaning or movement. The disease has its worst effects in the first three months of life. There is an incubation period of ten to fourteen days and the acute phase involves sneezing or snuffling. It is normally first seen in piglets of two to three weeks which can have a nasal discharge and conjunctivitis and tears can be produced. The chronic phase involves less frequent sneezing and a progressive deformity of the snout as defective growth of the bones round the nasal cavity produces a thickening of the snout, corrugation of the skin over the nose and protrusion of the lower incisors; the snout may also be drawn to one side. It is possible to treat sows and gilts to protect their progeny; this involves two injections with a six week interval between them. Bordetella bronchiseptica is a similar condition, affecting both the upper and lower respiratory tract.

Sunburn and Heatstroke

Sunburn is seldom a problem with rare breeds of pig as they generally have dark skins and coats, but pale skinned pigs such as the Middle White or the Welsh, when kept outdoors, can get sunburned, as can those with fine, sparser coats such as the Tamworth. Young pigs with tender skins can also get sunburned. Providing adequate shade and access to mud wallows is most helpful but if your pigs insist on sunning themselves to extreme, you might need to put some sun-cream on them or spray them afterwards with a soothing liquid.

Overheating can cause a disorder of the heat regulatory mechanism in the brain – loss of body heat is lessened and the pig's temperature can be raised to a dangerous degree, possibly over 43°C (110°F), and important nerve centres can become paralysed. Sunstroke involves high body temperature, whereas heat exhaustion has normal or low temperatures and loss of body water and salt. Pigs have small lung capacities compared with other domestic animals and they also have thick layers of fat which insulate their bodies and can interfere with loss of body heat. Their sweat glands are limited and so pigs lose very little water through their skin. Factors contributing to overheating are being confined in places with inadequate ventilation, having little shelter from the sun and being provided with too little water. Both temperature and humidity contribute to deaths from heatstroke. Sometimes pigs with early forms of heatstroke dip their backs in a peculiar manner and there is momentary paralysis of the hind-quarters. This characteristic symptom occurs once or twice a minute.

When overheated, pigs salivate a lot and frothy mucus can appear from their mouth and nose. If severe, blood can appear in this, indicating that the lungs have been affected. They also breathe very rapidly, opening their mouths to do so, have a fast and feeble pulse and can be very restless. They may be unable to get up and make convulsive movements or, if they can get to their feet, they may stagger in an uncoordinated way. To avoid overheating you can provide shade and wallows, feed in or near shady areas, ensure the animals have plenty of water and only move them in the cool parts of the day - avoiding parking in the sun (or even in the shade in extreme conditions of heat). Maintaining air movement through vehicles via air inlets at the side, pref-

erably at about snout level, is essential. Also, bedding in vehicles should be cut down and slightly dampened if the weather is very hot.

To treat overheating you need to act rapidly. If at a show, a minimum of bedding should be used and the earth of the pen should be soaked with cold water – even making a wallow if necessary. You can also continuously bath heads, legs, upper parts of their bodies and bellies in cool water either by sponging, spraying, or applying ice packs to their heads and legs until the body temperature starts to fall, but you should never throw a bucket of cold water over very hot animals as the shock could kill them. You can put suitable creams or lotions onto the affected skin to avoid blistering and soothe the hot sensation (both pharmaceutical and 'natural' products are available). You can also cool their floors with water or use fans to cool the air in their houses. Consult your vet urgently if the animals show significant signs of heatstroke. Symptoms of heatstroke can reappear after treatment is discontinued, so a check should be kept on any affected animals.

Mineral Deficiencies

This should not be a problem with most pigs kept in a traditional manner as, in addition to their specially formulated pig food, they will have access to soil that contains minerals. There are one or two minerals that can sometimes be in short supply, however, and it is worth looking out for any signs of deficiency. In particular, newly born piglets can sometimes become deficient in iron and some breeders give iron injections as a matter of routine. If this is done it needs to be given at three to four days of age. If, however, the piglets are given some earth to nibble on by putting a small turf in the creep area periodically – and later they are allowed free access to outside paddocks, this problem can be avoided or overcome and it is, in any case, less expensive and less stressful than injections that could carry a risk of introducing infection. I have never given my own piglets iron injections. Signs of anaemia can be hard to spot but include a yellowish or grey diarrhoea in young piglets, slow growth - with piglets appearing pale and hairy - and rapid respiration.

There is also a condition called 'thin sow syndrome,' which seems to involve a combination of parasite infection, cold and inadequate diet.

Swine Influenza/Pig Flu

This is an acute infectious respiratory disease. Symptoms include breathing problems, coughs, high temperatures and considerable weight loss. All animals in a herd tend to get it. There is no specific treatment for this illness apart from ensuring good bedding and a draught-free, dust-free environment and avoiding excessive movement. Recovery from this ailment tends to be rapid.

Transmissible Gastroenteritis (TGE) and Porcine Epidemic Diarrhoea (PED)

TGE is a very contagious disease with a short incubation period of up to three days. Symptoms include vomiting, severe diarrhoea, often watery with a greenish tinge and loss of appetite. There is a very high mortality rate in young piglets, especially those under two weeks old, although most weaned pigs recover well. PED tends to affect older pigs and diarrhoea is present but usually without the green tinge.

Joint-ill (Navel-ill)

This is an infection where organisms gain entrance through the navel or umbilicus, producing abscess formation at the site. The piglet fails to thrive which is usually the first sign. Subsequently, the disease can spread to the joints causing lameness. Piglets affected with this form of arthritis invariably die and abscesses may be found in the liver, lungs and kidney and there may also be peritonitis and pleurisy. The disease is associated with poor hygiene. To avoid this it is worth spraying the umbilical cords with antiseptic at birth. Farrowing in a clean and disinfected environment is also important as well as washing the sow with a mild antiseptic prior to putting her in the farrowing pen.

Erysipelas

The word means 'red skin' and the disease is caused by a bacterium - Erysipelothrix Rhusiopathiae - found in soil. Some healthy pigs can harbour this organism in their bone marrow and bowels and humans may acquire the disease through cuts or abrasions. There are four types of clinical signs for Erysipelas: peracute, acute, subacute and chronic.

Peracute Signs

Signs are non-existent – pigs are simply found dead with no symptoms.

Acute Signs

Acute signs appear suddenly and result in temperatures of 40°C (104°F) and above with death sometimes occurring within as little as a day or so. The animals withdraw from the herd, some lie down and show signs of depression and resent being disturbed. They have a stiff gait or lameness and shift their weight to ease the pain in their legs. They may shiver and/or vomit. Their heads are hung so that their backs are arched. They have a reduced appetite and may regurgitate their food.

Diamond-shaped, light pink to dark purple skin lesions appear and can be felt as raised welts (in some densely coated pigs the lesions are difficult to spot and identification is mainly through feeling the raised areas). If the lesions are light, they generally tend to disappear after a few days, whereas dark ones can precede chronic illness or death. When the animals recover the lameness may disappear or it may recur and become chronic. In suckling pigs there may be a fatal enteritis with yellowish or white, watery diarrhoea, often accompanied by septicaemia. This is quite infectious within litters but not so much between non-related groups in the same house. The coat becomes rough and the pigs become dehydrated and emaciated. Scouring pigs can re-infect themselves and help the organism to establish itself higher in the digestive tract, so frequent cleaning of pens is vital.

Subacute Signs

These signs are less severe, with Urticaria-like lesions of the skin that are dark red in colour, subsequently becoming paler.

Chronic Signs

Chronic signs follow the acute stage and can involve the loss of portions of skin (leaving scarring), or loss of parts of the ears, tail and feet, heart changes and arthritis/joint-swelling and lameness. Secondary infection also usually occurs. However, sometimes chronic illness is only diagnosed at post-mortem as there has been no history of illness.

Erysipelas is usually treated successfully with antibiotics but, to prevent it from occurring, you should vaccinate your piglets at around eight weeks of age and then a second time two weeks later and then every six months.

Parvovirus

This is a highly contagious, although not common, disease in pigs. It can cause sows to fail to come into season and there can also be a range of defects found in piglets – for example mummification, stillbirths and perinatal deaths (dying within two to three days of being born). The virus is spread via urine, faeces, semen, nasal secretions and afterbirths and can persist for months in the environment. It is possible to vaccinate prior to service and the virus can be killed in the environment by the use of common household bleach at a 1:30 dilution.

Swine Pox/Pig Pox

This is a viral infection transmitted by direct contact and is most common in the first four months of life and more serious in three to six week-old piglets. It is very mild in older piglets or pigs and is usually a relatively benign ailment, although it can be severe in some cases. The first signs are dullness and loss of appetite followed by small areas of reddening about half an inch in diameter on the skin of various parts of the body. Scab formation follows without the production of vesicles. The condition usually clears up in three weeks and treatment is not essential, however dressing of the raw surfaces after the scabs have been removed accelerates healing. The disease is infectious and as such sows with infected litters should be isolated and the pens thoroughly disinfected. External parasites can be associated with the infection, so measures should be taken to eliminate them. After recovery animals acquire immunity to the disease.

Leptospiral Infection

This is contracted from rats which harbour

the organisms in their kidneys and excrete them in their urine, contaminating food and water supplies. The disease can be taken up in mucous membranes such as in the mouth, or through skin abrasions and cuts. The disease particularly affects suckling piglets of one to two months old. They show listlessness, a lack of appetite and a high temperature of 40.5° to 41°C (105° to 106°F) for two to three days and then develop jaundice which, over twenty four hours, extends over the whole body. Death usually occurs at that stage although some may recover. Abortions can also occur together with stillbirths and fever, loss of milk and jaundice in sows. Injections of antibiotics can treat the disease if given early and vaccination can also be used before service or in young piglets (before six to ten weeks of age).

Ringworm

The organism that produces ringworm lives in the soil and can exist there for long periods. It produces spots that enlarge to cover wide areas. The spots are usually about four to six centimetres in diameter, reddish to light brown and slightly roughened, but not obviously raised. The symptoms often occur behind the ears and spread to the neck. Itching tends to occur and dry crusts may be formed and hair tends to fall out. However, a heavy coat may obscure the lesions.

Urticaria (Nettlerash)

This is a skin condition that tends to be seen in young pigs more than in piglets or adults. Small red pimples appear on the skin, usually on the belly, sides and inside the thighs. Mostly it is a mild condition but in some cases an infection can set in, causing chronic dermatitis and skin thickening. Usually no treatment is necessary, although it can help to put soothing cream on the affected areas.

Arthritis/Rheumatism

Pigs can be susceptible to bone and joint problems, especially if they are kept in cold, damp conditions. For this reason wooden floors are preferable to concrete or earth. Affected pigs have stiffness and find it difficult to get up or walk and may spend much of their time lying down. The joints can become swollen and often the pigs are worse in winter than in summer because of the adverse weather conditions. While arthritis/rheumatism are unlikely to be totally curable, warm housing, massaging in creams that heat up the skin or the application of anti-inflammatory products (pharmaceutical or 'natural') can give relief from the symptoms. Undue stress to the joints should be avoided, so pigs that are in this kind of condition should probably not be bred from as pregnancy would put too much extra weight on the limbs and joints.

Bowel Oedema

This is caused by a bacterium and is stress-related. It occurs in newly weaned pigs – usually eight to fourteen weeks and occasionally in older pigs. It is characterised by staggering and usually - but not always - swollen eyelids. If you see these symptoms you should seek advice from your vet. The cause is usually a change to a rich diet or possibly ingesting some poisonous material. Sudden diet changes should be avoided and, if bowel oedema is present, food should usually be restricted or withheld for twelve hours and re-introduced slowly.

Poisoning

Although this is rare you should be careful not to expose pigs to substances such as Warfarin, insecticides, herbicides or lead. These can be fatal, although some treatment may be possible. You should also take care to avoid mouldy feeds which can ferment in the gut and may sometimes be fatal, and also poisonous plants such as ragwort.

Teeth, Tusks and Feet

On the whole pigs are unlikely to need much attention to their mouths or feet. One exception to this are boars whose tusks can grow long and become sharp and potentially dangerous. If this happens their tusks can be trimmed using a wire saw that cuts through them, or by using cutters. Cutters can, however, result in jagged ends and the wire saw is usually better.

Animals kept on very soft ground or allowed to become overweight may sometimes have overgrown feet. Pigs' feet keep on growing and if they have some hard ground to walk on they are able to keep their feet from becoming excessively long. If feet do become too long they can be trimmed back using foot clippers.

It may be necessary to confine or sedate animals that need to have their mouths or feet dealt with. If they are sedated, ensure this is carried out by a competent person and that the animals are not allowed to lie on a cold surface while sedated as they can become chilled (covering with straw helps).

It is also important to ensure that your pigs don't have problems with loose or decaying teeth, as this can be painful and affect their eating. Any pig off its food, with no other signs, should have its teeth checked in case they are the cause of the trouble.

Notifiable Diseases in the UK

There are some diseases that are 'notifiable,' which means that, if you suspect signs of the disease, you must immediately notify the Defra Divisional Veterinary Manager at your local Animal Health Divisional Office. The notifiable diseases are:

Classical Swine Fever

This is a contagious disease that last occurred in the UK in 2000. It has acute and chronic forms and is spread to pigs by infected pigs, pig meat, dirty vehicles, boots etc. It enters the pig through ingestion or inhalation. In the mild and chronic forms of the disease, the signs are less obvious. There may be a short-lived lack of appetite and a fever and possibly abortion. However, in the acute form pigs are very dull and off their food with a high fever of 40°C to 41°C (106 to 107°F). They may cough and initially show constipation then, later, diarrhoea. There may be a discharge from the eyes and nose and the skin may become reddened and blotchy. Pregnant sows may abort or give birth to a weak litter. Some newborn piglets have tremors. The pigs do not walk straight but sway, and their legs may cross. Some can die within two to three days of the viral infection, while others may survive this phase but then go on to develop lung complications.

African Swine Fever (ASF)

This is similar to Classical Swine Fever but is caused by a different virus. It can be given to pigs by ticks and biting flies as well as directly from infected pigs and pig meat. There are acute and chronic forms of ASF. In the acute disease, pigs firstly go off their food and are extremely dull with a high temperature (40° to 42°C/104°to 108°F). They can then have diarrhoea, vomiting, coughing and a purple blotching of the skin. They may have a swaying gait, abort their litters and have a discharge from the eyes and nose. African Swine Fever has never occurred in the UK to date.

Foot and Mouth Disease (FMD)

A major outbreak occurred in the UK in 2001 and, to a lesser degree, again in 2007. It is a highly infectious viral disease affecting pigs and other ruminating animals. The incubation period is between two and ten days. The chief symptom in pigs is sudden lameness. There is also a fever of up to 41°C (106°F) or more as well as eruptions on the skin and mucous membranes. Mouth symptoms are not usually visible, but blisters may develop on the snout or on the tongue and along the udder. Affected animals refuse food, lose condition and prefer to lie down and, when made to move, squeal loudly and hobble painfully, though lameness may not be so obvious where the pigs are on deep bedding or soft ground. The blisters form on the upper edge of the hoof, where the skin and horn meet, and on the heels and in the cleft. They may extend right round the hoof head, with the result that the horn becomes detached. Once the lesions erupt, the pig's temperature falls rapidly and symptoms of acute disturbance fade. Within two to three days the animal regains appetite and begins recovering. Eventually new horn starts to grow and the old hoof is carried down and finally shed. This process resembles the loss of a fingernail following some blow or other injury.

Swine Vesicular Disease (SVD)

This last occurred in Great Britain in 1982. The symptoms are clinically indistinguishable from FMD but SVD only affects pigs. There is a fever of up to 41°C (106°F), then vesicles (blisters) develop on the coronary band, typically at the junction with the heel. The disease usually appears suddenly but does not spread with the same rapidity as FMD. Mortality is low but, in acute cases, there can be some loss of production. Lameness develops due to the eruption of vesicles at the top of the hooves and between the toes. Vesicles may also develop on the snout, tongue and lips. The surface under the vesicles is red and this gradually changes colour as healing develops. The entire hoof may be shed. In less severe cases, the healed lesion may grow down the hoof and this is seen by a black transverse mark. Recovery is usually complete within two to three weeks.

Aujeszky's Disease

Aujeszky's disease is also caused by a virus and last occurred in Great Britain in 1989. It is, as yet, still not entirely eliminated in Ireland. Affected pigs show a variety of signs including sneezing, coughing, laboured breathing and fever. They may show nervous signs too, such as trembling, circling and a swaying gait. Pregnant sows might abort or give birth to stillborn or mummified litters. Deaths are highest in younger pigs.

Teschen Disease (Porcine Enterovirus Encephalomyelitis)

This has never occurred in the UK. Initially, infected pigs have a fever and a loss of appetite, are dull and slightly uncoordinated. As the disease progresses there is irritability, stiffness, muscular tremors or rigidity and convulsions. There may also be grinding of the teeth, smacking of the lips and squealing, as if in pain. The voice may change or be lost entirely. The course of the disease is usually acute and death, generally preceded by paralysis, normally occurs within three to four days of the appearance of symptoms. Mildly affected animals may recover. All age groups of pig are susceptible to this disease. (A milder form of this disease is called Talfan disease, and this has occurred in the UK).

Vesicular Stomatitis

This is a very rare disease of pigs which has never occurred in the UK, but can also affect cattle, horses and people. This disease, like SVD and FMD, causes blisters, but a different virus is involved. Areas of skin become blanched, followed by the formation of vesicles on the snout, lips, tongue, hard and soft palate and the coronary band. Lesions may also occur in some other areas of the skin, especially where there is abrasion of tissue. The vesicles yield a fluid as they burst, usually six to twenty four hours after formation. The hoof may become detached if vesicles have gathered there. Mortality rates are moderate to low.

Anthrax

This last occurred in the UK in 2002 and is an acutely infectious disease caused by bacterial infection. Pigs are more resistant to this than other farm animals. Infection has been caused by the presence of spores in foodstuffs that have been contaminated with animal products. Spores can also live for some time in slurry and contaminated housing. Symptoms can include high temperature and fluid-filled swellings around the neck, diarrhoea and sudden death can occur. This is a notifiable disease that can be transmitted to people. Treatment is by antibiotics but animals are usually found dead.

Rabies

This was eradicated in the UK in 1922. It is spread by saliva from affected animals. Symptoms include paralysis and aggression.

PMWS (Post-Weaning Multi-Systemic Wasting Syndrome)
PDNS (Porcine Dermatitis and Nephropathy Syndrome)

The following information comes from the Meat and Livestock Commission's booklets:

These are two relatively new, inter-related diseases that are a significant threat to the world-wide pig industries. PMWS was first recognised in Canada in 1996 (and retrospectively diagnosed in 1985). It was first identified in the UK in 1999. PDNS also emerged as a major problem for pig farmers at the same time as PMWS appeared, although it is now believed that the first cases of PDNS were seen in 1993, and possibly even earlier.

The causes of both PMWS and PDNS are not fully understood, but research has identified that an infectious agent - Porcine Circovirus Type 2 (PCV2) – plays a significant role in both diseases. PCV2 is widespread and found in both healthy and diseased pigs.

The virus is extremely resistant to heat and most disinfectants and its presence can be confirmed in most healthy herds, and all diseased herds, by the presence of circulating antibodies. This means that the presence of the virus does not necessarily lead to disease. On its own, the virus can cause very mild disease, but its incidence and severity is greatly increased when pigs are also infected by another virus or their immune system is challenged by other agents – this suggests that a trigger is needed to cause disease. The virus also appears to spread easily and, although there is a lack of understanding in this area, it is likely that this can take place through:

• Mechanical transfer via dung, manure on boots, equipment, vehicles and animals etc.
• The carrier pig. The virus can persist in

infected pigs for up to six months and is excreted via the nose, faeces and semen, meaning that the spread can take place by direct pig-to-pig contact.
• Semen. It can be excreted for up to six weeks in semen so it is theoretically possible that it could be spread by AI or natural matings, although to date this has not been confirmed.

Key points to understand about PMWS are:

• Symptoms of PMWS can vary considerably from farm to farm and in its early stages it can be confused with other diseases. Symptoms include the appearance of red/brown lesions under the skin, with haemorrhages, usually appearing on the ears, face, flanks, legs and hams.
• Mortality rates from PMWS are also variable.
• It can strike any herd regardless of its health status and production system.
• The onset of the disease is often slow and it generally affects pigs between six to sixteen weeks old, although it can affect pigs from five to twenty four weeks and the age of affected pigs seems to be increasing.
• It causes lack of appetite, wasting, depression and death.
• Mild conjunctivitis with tear-staining is often seen.
• Affected pigs look pale and/or jaundiced and have diarrhoea.
• Sick pigs show severe respiratory distress.
• Sudden death of good pigs is sometimes the only symptom.
• The number of pigs affected can range from 3% to 50%.
• Up to 80% of affected pigs die.
• Secondary diseases such as pneumonia and meningitis are common.
• PMWS is often seen after an official outbreak of PDNS and vice-versa.

Some Other key Facts About the PCV2 Virus:

• Its severity appears to be related to levels of infectious agents on the farm.
• Continuous production systems challenge the immune system, enabling the virus to invade the lymph system.
• Poor nutrition predisposes animals to it.
• Certain breeds may be more susceptible.
• Disease is not seen in sows, gilts and suckling pigs, although some reproduction problems have been reported.
• Pigs with high levels of colostral antibody do not appear to succumb to disease once colostrum intake stops (after the first twenty four hours) as the immunity status of the piglets is fixed.
• Piglets can be infected in the uterus or at birth.
• The better the health status of the herd, the less severe the disease outbreak is.

Recommendations for avoiding the effects of PMWS and PDNS include four 'golden rules:'

Limiting pig-to-pig contact: This includes both direct contact and indirect via people, manure or surgical instruments. (Author's note: although these are the guidelines given, there is also an argument that allowing all pigs on one holding to be in contact with each other at some stage ensures a common exposure, and antibody development, to disease. While guidelines are relevant for large scale pig production, small producers may wish to take different measures in this respect, allowing their pigs more 'social' contact while being aware of any possible risks this could expose them to).

Avoiding stress: Consider any activity that could be stressful and whether it could be done in a less stressful manner. Avoid excessive mixing of pigs. Also avoid exposing pigs to chilling draughts which can cause problems.

Maintaining good hygiene: Cleaning, disinfecting, good hygiene and bio-security are vital. It is important to use less intensive systems of production and keep pigs in small groups. Also, treating sows and gilts for parasites before they enter the farrowing house can help maintain good condition and thereby good colostrum levels.

Maintaining good nutrition: This is important both for growth and for development of the immune system. Piglets should get considerable amounts of colostrum (first milk from their mothers) during their first twelve hours of life. High quality diets later on with high levels of antioxidants will also strengthen the immune system.

No specific conventional treatments have been identified as wholly effective, but antibiotics can help, as can some corticosteroid injections. Piglets can also be treated with serum, although this must be discussed with your vet.

Research on this topic is currently being carried out at various institutes and a vaccine is under development, but is not yet available. Further information can be found at the Meat and Livestock Commission website (www. bpex.org.uk).

PMWS and PDNS are not included in the tables section as they are very difficult to categorise and thanfully rare.

Natural Treatment Methods

Although licensed medication is the conventional course adopted for prevention and treatment of ill health in pigs, there are alternatives. Increasingly, people are turning to 'natural' remedies and finding they give excellent results. It is worth remembering that many pharmaceutical products originated from natural sources; aspirin, for example, originally came from Willow bark.

Most vets will automatically use conventional medication, but many are using other kinds of treatment, either alongside, or instead of pharmaceuticals; for example, homeopathy and healing. Some alternative remedies are debatable, but the use of others is proven, in many cases with clinical trials.

Aloe Vera

One type of natural remedy that is particularly effective in animal treatment is Aloe Vera. It is a plant that grows in hot, dry conditions, with many of the plants originating from Africa. It is a member of the lily family and related to other medicinal plants such as onions and garlic, although it looks like a cactus. The most commonly used Aloe plant is Aloe Barbadensis Miller, which has some of the most potent medical properties.

Aloe Vera gel, the sticky substance found in the middle of the leaves of the plant, contains at least seventy five known ingredients including vitamins, minerals, amino acids and enzymes; it has two applications:
• It works on the immune system
• It works on epithelial tissue (external skin and internal body linings such as the gut, the lining of the nose, the inside of the mouth, the lungs and so forth)

Some of the actions of Aloe Vera are to:
• Increase cell-division and healing - wounds treated with Aloe generally heal at least a third faster than with conventional veterinary preparations because Aloe increases cell division by fibroblasts in the skin by at least three times - making more fibre

• Improve blood flow to the skin through capillary dilation
• Act as a natural local anaesthetic
• Act as a natural anti-inflammatory agent
• Kill certain bacteria, viruses, fungi and yeasts
• Act as an antioxidant
• Act as a natural cleaner and moisturiser
• Feed basal cells to keep skin healthy and looking good
• Decrease itching
• Decrease bleeding through encouraging coagulation when applied to minor wounds such as a graze
• Lower body temperature (probably due to its content of salicylic acid content, an aspirin-like agent) and take the heat out of inflammatory skin conditions

Aloe is also an adaptogen, which means that the body takes out of the gel what it needs to help the condition from which it is suffering – in other words it helps to restore balance. Animals on Aloe typically have thicker, shinier and better quality coats and appear brighter and more full of life. There are no known side effects in the use of stabilised Aloe Vera products and Aloe is safe to use in conjunction with other veterinary drugs and often enhances their action, for example antibiotics and homeopathic remedies.

Pigs also seem to like Aloe and, although it works best when taken on an empty stomach, it may be hard to get the pigs to take it without a little bit of food. I find that pouring it onto a slice of bread is a good way to give it to them. Some of the conditions that you can use Aloe for in pigs are:
• Arthritis
• Dry skin
• Scouring
• Constipation
• Cuts and other small wounds
• Cleaning udders
• Greasy pig disease
• Sunburn
• Insect bites
• Mastitis

It is important to use products that have a high level of Aloe in them. The most beneficial results appear to come from cold stabilised gel – a product that has not been boiled or filtered – as these processes appear to interfere with the synergistic properties of the Aloe. Synergism is where substances work together to produce an effect greater than the sum of their individual effects – the presence of the various elements in the gel enhancing the action of each of the others. Do remember that Aloe will not treat all conditions and, as with other natural treatment methods, Aloe tends to be slower acting than pharmaceutical compounds. So some conditions - especially acute ones -will need conventional medication, although it may be that using Aloe to accompany medication can help the animal to recover more quickly and in a more natural way. In his book, 'Aloe Vera, Nature's Gift (Aloe Vera in Veterinary Practice),' David Urch recommends that pigs of 150kg (330lb) receive a treatment dose of 120ml of Aloe Vera drinking gel a day, or a maintenance dose/general tonic of 30ml a day.

Acidotherapy

Another treatment method I have been told about, although I have not used it, is Acidotherapy. The principle behind this is that pathogens need alkalinity in order to survive, whereas beneficial bacteria need an acidic medium. High levels of ammonia, found in urine, create a high pH environment (low acidity/ high alkalinity), which is ideal for the spread of respiratory disease; bedding too can also be very alkaline. Acidotherapy treatment involves spraying (or 'fogging') an area with a diluted acid solution (organic acids, blended with aromatic oils and then diluted with warm water) in order to produce surfaces that are fatal to pathogens (and also helping keep dust levels down). It is also suggested that the spraying is done while animals are in the area, so that they ingest the air that is being treated. This apparently clears the animal's airways, helping with breathing problems and clearing the lungs from mucus - and works very effectively on ailments such as rhinitis.

General health facts

A pig's normal heart-beat ranges from 200 to 280 beats per minute in newborn piglets, 70 to 80 in young adults at rest and 70 to 110 in adults generally. Heart rate is increased by pregnancy, feeding and excitement and decreases with increasing body weight.

The respiratory rate in resting pigs varies from 10 to 30 per minute (50 in very young piglets) and increases with very high temperatures.

Body temperature ranges from 38 to 40°C with a mean of 38.8°C (101.5 to 104°F with a mean of 102°F). High external temperatures can affect body temperature, especially in heavier pigs. The body temperature of piglets falls at birth and then recovers, as in humans. If exposed to chilling temperatures the adult value is not reached for several days instead of on the first day. New born piglets are relatively tolerant to hypothermia, but under such conditions develop a very low blood glucose concentration and may also manifest blood thinning.

On the whole pigs don't sweat. A little water may be lost from the skin but this is relatively slight.

The greatest weight gain, and most efficient feed utilisation, occurs at an average ambient temperature of 24°C (75°F) for pigs of 32-65kg (70-143lb) and 15.5°C (60°F) for ones of 65-120kg (143-264lb).

Giving injections

If you are going to give injections to your pigs, you should get your vet to show you how to do this. Injections are generally given either into the muscle (intramuscular) or under the skin (subcutaneous). When injecting pigs they should be restrained, either in a crush pen (one that is only just bigger than the animal, so that it cannot turn around or climb over) or by a snare that goes over its snout. Unexpected movements can result in the needle breaking or coming out so that the product sprays outside the pig, injures the pig or the handler or is injected at the wrong site. All injection equipment needs to be clean and sterile (and preferably new) before use and needles need to be sharp and of the correct size – smaller for small pigs and piglets, but if they are too thin there is a danger that they will bend or break. On the whole, pigs of up to 10kg (22lb) need a 1.5 to 2cm (½ to ¾ in) needle for intra-muscular injection, 10 to 30kg (22 to 66lb) need 2 to 2.5cm (¾ to 1in), 25 to 30kg (55 to 66lb) need 2.5 to 3cm (1 to 1¼ in) and over 100kg (220lb), 4 to 4.5 cm (1½ to 1¾ in). If the product is injected into fat rather than muscle there will be a slow uptake and a poor response to it, so correct angles of injection are important. Incorrect procedures can result in lumps or abscesses at the injection site, so good technique is vital.

Stopping contamination

It is worth keeping available some strong disinfectant and a large, shallow container to fill with water and disinfectant so that, if you have one pig with an ailment, you can dip your boots into the disinfectant before entering another pig's area. You should change your gloves or dip them into the disinfectant too as a safety precaution against contamination.

If you have a pig that is ill, or a new one that has just arrived from elsewhere, or that has returned from a show, the vet or a mating, it is helpful to isolate it temporarily so that the likelihood of infection being transmitted is reduced. For this purpose you should have a pig house that the pig can occupy on its own, or at least an area with double fencing, so that pigs can not actually touch each other through a fence. There are specific isolation regulations in some of the health and welfare legislation and a twenty day isolation period is the norm.

Record keeping

Under The Welfare of Farmed Animals (England) Regulations 2000 it is necessary to keep records of medical treatments given to animals, including which animals were treated, the date they were treated, the name of the product, the quantity of medicine used, the date treatment finished, the date any withdrawal period ends and the name of the person who administered the medicine. You can also record the batch number of the medicine used, although this is not strictly a legal requirement. And if there are any mortalities these should also be recorded. Records must be completed within seventy two hours of administration and must be kept for at least three years from the date on which the medication was given or the date of an inspection. It is, of course, worth recording for your own information any kind of treatment given to your animals, whether pharmaceutical or other. You can obtain pre-printed Record of Treatment books from various places including the Pig Veterinary Society. It is also worth keeping records of when medicines were acquired and disposed of.

Disposing of medical waste

All needles, syringes, remnants of drugs and so forth should be disposed of correctly. Old and part-used POM products are classified as 'special waste' under current waste legislation. This means that disposal has to be via a licensed waste management contractor, preferably to an incinerator. Your local Environment Agency office will have details of all local approved Waste Management Contractors. PML, P and GSL products and their empty containers may or may not be classified as 'special waste.' If in doubt about disposal, check with your vet or contact the manufacturer, supplier or local Environment Agency office. Be especially careful when handling sharp needles.

Withdrawal times

All licensed medicines have 'withdrawal periods.' This means that for a period after the use of such products an animal cannot be used for food production. The withdrawal period is generally twenty eight days for meat animals and seven days for milked animals. You should check this and record it in your medicine book for each product administered. If you are planning to send animals for slaughter you must be careful about any medication you give them in the period beforehand, including pour-on anti-parasite preparations, antibiotics, vaccinations and so forth. Non-pharmaceutical, 'natural' products (such as Aloe Vera) do not have withdrawal periods as they are not classified as medicines. If you are registered as organic, however, even the use of natural products may need to be declared and included in your health and welfare plan.

Finding a vet

Choose your vet carefully. Not all practices specialise in treating 'large animals' and few nowadays have specialist expertise in pig health, as the pig industry has changed so much. In some areas there are veterinary practices that do work a lot with pigs, but these tend to be in areas that have large, intensive, pig production units. Check what knowledge the veterinary practice has of pig treatment before deciding which one to use and ask other local pig keepers whom they would recommend before deciding.

Disposal of dead animals

Under recent legislation (2003), routine burial and burning of animal carcasses on farms and smallholdings is no longer permitted. Carcasses have to be disposed of according to new regulations and the National Fallen Stock Company can give you information on these.

DIAGNOSTIC GUIDE TO PIG AILMENTS AND TREATMENT

Signs of Disease	Causes	Treatment and Prevention
HEAD AND FACE		
Discharge from the eyes.	Slight discharge not uncommon in short nosed breeds.	No action.
	Dusty environment causing irritation to eye membranes.	Improve ventilation and change bedding.
	Conjunctivitis due to bacterial infection; often sequel to bad ventilation.	Antibiotic eye ointment or drops.
	Rhinitis unlikely cause in adults as affected pigs not used for breeding.	Cull any clinically affected animalsl from herd.
Eyes dull and lifeless.	Part of any general disease.	Check for other symptoms before attempting diagnosis or treatment.
Membranes of the eye pale or white.	Anaemia due to internal parasites (gut or stomach worms), or internal haemorrhage caused by stomach ulcers.	Dose with anthelmintic. Difficult to treat, supportive treatment only.
Membranes of the eye yellow.	Jaundice usually the result of bacterial infection eg. Leptospira or fungus eg. Aspergillus (NB. both infectious to people).	Antibiotic. Check water supply for cleanliness. Rodent control. Feed is likely source of fungus/check.
Eyes sunk into sockets.	Dehydration usually as the result of vomiting and/or scouring.	Electrolytes as fluid replacement. Other treatment may be indicated when a diagnosis is made.
Nasal discharge with sneezing.	Dusty environment.	Improve ventilation and get rid of dust.
	Atrophic Rhinitis or Inclusion Body Rhinitis are diseases of young pigs.	Any adult animals with twisted snouts should be culled from the herd and not bred from.
	Upper respiratory infection by virus or bacteria.	Antibiotic may be required for treatment.
Salivation.	Sores in mouth or on tongue due to bacterial infection following an injury or bad tooth. Possible tumour (rare).	Further investigation may be needed. Treat with antibiotic. Euthanasia on welfare grounds in case of tumour.
Salivation with sores in mouth and on snout.	Consider possibility of Foot and Mouth disease or Swine Vesicular Disease (NB. both are virus diseases and notifiable).	If there is any suspicion of either of these two diseases you must get veterinary advice ASAP.
Itching and skin thickening around and between the eyes.	Mange due to infection by Sarcoptes scabiei mite.	Topical or injectable ectoparasiticides.
EARS		
One or both ears swollen.	Common cause is abscess or haematoma (blood blister).	Lance and drain abscess. Leave haematoma alone if possible as blood will be absorbed over a few weeks. In both cases it will be better to isolate the patient over the acute period.

Signs of Disease	Causes	Treatments and Prevention
EARS CONTINUED		
Brown discharge from one or both ears with some irritation.	Mange due to Sarcoptes scabiei. Common.	As above. Topical ectoparasiticides or injectable Ivermectin.
Red discolouration of both ears.	If healthy outdoor pig, sunburn.	Provide shade and mud wallows.
Blue or purple discolouration of both ears.	Terminal stage of many different diseases eg. Blue Ear disease or Salmonella (NB. could be infectious to people) etc. Heart failure.	Pig is actuely ill. Get vet ASAP. Poor prognosis. Need vet ASAP.
SKIN		
Skin itchy with brown discharge on back around eyes and ears and on legs.	Mange due to Sarcoptes scabiei.	As above. Treat with topical eg. Porect or injectable eg. Ivermectin ectoparasiticide. Treat and move to clean accommodation. Eradicate by treating every 10 days.
Skin itching without discharge.	Check for lice (Haematopinus suis).	Topical or injectable ectoparasiticide.
Skin with generalised redness, especially the ears.	If otherwise healthy and outdoors this is sunburn.	Provide shade and mud wallows.
Skin with red raised sores, usually diamond shape along back.	Swine Erysipelas, chronic form of infection by Erysipelothrix insodiosa.	Penicillin is still the most effective treatment. Vaccination is highly effective.
Skin with purple discolouration of ears and belly.	May be the terminal sign of any toxic or septicaemic disease but consider in particular Salmonella (NB. could be infectious to people) or, if just farrowed, acute Metritis.	Get vet ASAP. Will need to check for other symptoms to make a diagnosis before treament is started.
BREATHING		
Rapid breathing.	Stress due to pain or hyperthermia or over exercise. Pneumonia due to virus, bacteria of lungworm (Metastrongylus apri) infection. Swine flu is a common virus infection, Pasteurella and Haemophilus are common bacterial infections. Consider chronic heart failure if pig is old and overweight.	Identify and remove source of stress. If hyperthermic douse with cold water. Sedatives may be useful. Antibiotic by injection or in feed or in water. Anthelmintic for lungworm. Get vet to check diagnosis and environment for adequate ventilation. Difficult to treat and poor prognosis. Vet may try cardiac and respiratory stimulants and diuretics if there is fluid retention.

Signs of Disease	Causes	Treatment and Prevention
BREATHING CONTINUED		
Shallow Breathing.	Probably asleep. Possibly in terminal stage of illness but there would be other symptoms. Some pigs with high temperatures eg. with Erysipelas will lie very still.	No action - let sleeping pigs lie. Check for other symptoms. Check temperature before treating. If in doubt get the vet.
Coughing.	Respiratory disease/see above for Pneumonia.	See above.
Sporadic dry cough in outdoor pigs.	Likely cause is lungworm or migrating roundworm.	Oral or injectable anthelmintic. Move to clean pasture. Pasture may need resting or cultivating for some years to be rid of the parasite.
TEMPERATURE (normal range is 101.5 - 102.5°F)		
Raised.	Often the result of infection by bacteria or virus. Pigs are very susceptible to hyperthermia in hot weather. Pain or stress can cause a mild fever.	Further investigation required before treatment. Apply cold water. A sedative may be useful. Identify source of stress. Analgesic for pain.
Lowered.	Check again. If temperature is 2-3 degress lower than normal the pig may be terminally ill.	Check again for other symptoms. If in doubt get the vet.
Sweating.	Pigs do not appear to sweat.	Hot pigs lose heat through the skin. They pant and use water and mud to cool off.
Shivering.	See above for lowered temperature but probably not serious.	Thin sows often shiver to raise body temperature. They have difficulty keeping warm in cold weather. Insulate and weatherproof housing.
DUNG		
Constipation.	Quite common in sows before and after farrowing.	Liquid paraffin in the food or drinking water. Bran either in feed or as a mash. Vegetables and grass can be useful.
Scouring, without blood.	Some virus infections are common eg. Epidemic Diarrhoea and T.G.E. Parasitism due to bowel worms eg. Strongyles or whipworms.	No vaccine available. Most adults will self-cure. Make sure they have plentiful access to fresh drinking water. Regular worming with anthelmintic and good hygiene.
Scouring with blood.	Bacterial infection eg. Salmonella. (NB. could be infectious to people) or Swine Dysentery at times of stress eg. farrowing.	Antibiotic treatment and hygiene is vital. Tiamutin and Lincocin are drugs of choice for treatment of Dysentery.
Vomiting.	Gastritis as the result of overeating or eating something unsuitable or stomach worms or stress resulting in ulceration of the stomach wall. Virus infections eg. Epidemic Diarrhoea or T.G.E.	Remove unsuitable diet and give fluids only for 24-36 hours. If suspect stomach worms, dose with anthelmintic. Adult pigs will self-cure providing they have plenty to drink.

Signs of Disease	Causes	Treatment and Prevention
DUNG CONTINUED		
Abdominal distension without pain.	Ascites ie. Dropsy as the result of heart or liver failure.	Difficult to treat, poor prognosis. Diuretics may be helpful.
	Peritonitis usually as a result of stomach or bowel ulceration.	Difficult to treat. Antibiotic may be helpful if early in disease.
	Abdominal tumour.	Euthanasia on welfare grounds.
Abdominal distention with pain.	Stomach or intestinal torsion.	Euthanasia on welfare grounds.
	Outdoor pigs might have a fluke infection.	Fluke anthelmintic and avoid ill drained pasture where the snail is the intermediate host for the parasite.
Abdominal distention with blood or pus in urine.	Cystitis and pus in the kidneys (Pyelonephritis). Can be painful although abdominal distention may not be too apparent.	Antibiotic, particularly in early stages. May be necessary to cull chronic cases.
INFERTILITY - FEMALE		
Failure to come into season.	Hormone imbalance or failure. This may be inherited or due to faulty nutrition or management.	Hormone therapy may be helpful. Check diet, sow may be too thin or too fat. Keep animal within sound, sight and smell of boar.
	May be pregnant.	Check.
	Vitamin deficiency eg. vitamin A or Biotin.	Feed analysis may be useful to check for deficiency. Inclusion of vitamin supplements in the ration.
	Failure to notice when in season. Heat period in the winter may be short.	Improve management.
Irregular heat periods. Normal cycle is every 21 days.	Cystic ovaries due to hormone imbalance.	Hormone injections may be helpful.
	Infectious infertility/virus eg. Smedi/Parvo/bacterial disease eg. Erysipelas, Leptospirosis (NB. infectious to people).	Needs careful investigation by vet. blood tests and swabs most helpful. Depending on cause, vaccines and antibiotic may be used to treat. Management also has large contribution to make.
ABORTION		
	General virus disease with other symptoms eg. Swine fever, Aujesky's Disease or Blue Ear Disease (NB. Swine Fever and Aujesky's Disease are notifiable diseases).	Blood tests required for diagnosis. Check on current status of Blue Ear disease. No treatment available.
	Specific virus diseases eg. Parvo virus or Smedi infections.	Vaccine available for Parvo infections, not for Smedi. Try to infect susceptible stock before pregnancy.
	Bacterial infection eg. Swine Erysipelas and Leptospirosis (NB. infectious to people).	Vaccine a must against Erysipelas. Antibiotic, hygiene and rodent control used against Leptospirosis.

Signs of Disease	Causes	Treatment and Prevention
ABORTION CONTINUED		
Vaginal discharge. Clear discharge with or without blood stain.	If pregnant may be about to give birth. Slight discharge may be apparent when in season.	Get experienced help to check if in doubt. If in season there should be other behavioural signs.
Purulent smelly discharge sometimes with straining after farrowing.	Metritis ie. infection in the genital tract with or without retained piglets or afterbirth.	Check for piglets and afterbirth and remove where possible. Antibiotic by injection and in pessaries or irrigation. Job for the vet.
Discharge without straining after farrowing.	Farrowing Fever syndrome ie. after farrowing when the udder is inflamed and little or no milk is produced. Specific infection eg. Blue Ear Disease (NB. check current status of disease).	Antibiotic, corticosteroids and oxytocin may be helpful. Make sure that sow is not over fed and constipated before farrowing. No specific treatment.
INFERTILITY - MALE		
	Deficiency diseases eg. vitamin A causes lack of libido. Orthopaedic problems eg. sore back, legs or pelvis.	Either vitamin A injections or nutritional supplement. Get vet to check and treat any lameness.
MASTITIS		
All glands affected, red, sore and painful.	Acute bacterial infection causing Metritis.	Antibiotic, corticosteroids and oxytocin. Improve hygiene, clip piglets' teeth. Vaccination may be helpful in some cases.
Less acute syndrome with vaginal discharge and failure to let down milk.	Farrowing Fever due to variety of bacterial infections. Constipation may be a factor.in the syndrome.	Antibiotic etc. as for Mastitis. Massage the udder with udder cream. Prevent constipation by cutting down on feed prior to farrowing and make up balance with bran or give liquid paraffin.
Lack of milk after farrowing without animal being ill.	Lack of mammary development in immature gilts. Premature farrowing. Failure of milk let down.	Milk may come after a few hours. Milk may come after a few hours. Oxytocin injection will bring almost immediate results.
Only one or two glands swollen and sore.	Mastitis (see above).	Treat as for generalised Mastitis. If animal has glands that are still hard and swollen after piglets are weaned then cull the sow.

Signs of Disease	Causes	Treatment and Prevention
LAMENESS		
FEET		
Swelling around the base of one or more claws.	Septic joints in the feet. Common. Many due to poor flooring causing damage to the sole allowing infection to penetrate.	Antibiotic must be given as soon as lesions are seen. Chronic abscesses may require surgery. Get vet to check flooring.
	Biotin deficiency may also predispose to foot infections.	Biotin supplement in feed.
Blisters around and between base of claws.	Virus infections cause blisters and lameness ie. Foot and Mouth disease and Swine Vesicular disease (NB. both notifiable diseases).	Check for blisters in mouth and snout and if suspicious contact your vet.
General foot soreness without obvious lesions.	Laminitis ie. inflammation in the foot due to overfeeding or Toxaemia after farrowing.	Pain killers and antibiotic if appropriate. Reduce feed and add more roughage.
LIMBS		
	Injury eg. fracture, nerve damage, puncture wounds and strains.	All but the most minor will need some veterinary attention.
Swollen, painful joints.	Non-septic arthritis caused by trauma to the joint.	Pain killing, corticosteroids and non-steroidal anti-inflammatory drugs can all be used. Animal may have to be culled.
	Swine Erysipelas can cause non-septic arthritis.	Treat early in the disease to prevent arthritis. Once arthritis is present antibiotic may have little value. All adult animals **must** be vaccinated twice a year.
	Septic arthritis ie. pus in the joint(s) due to a variety of bacteria.	Early treatment with an antibiotic that can cross the joint membrane barrier is vital. eg. ampicillin. Prognosis is poor.
Hind leg paralysis ie. unable to stand.	Usually some form of pelvic or spinal injury, often before or after farrowing.	Pain killing drugs, corticosteroids and non-steroidal anti-inflammatory drugs may all be helpful. Soft deep bedding and good nursing. If no response in a few days, euthanasia on welfare grounds.
	Spinal abscess often after tail biting.	No treatment. Euthanasia on welfare grounds.
BEHAVIOUR		
Loss of appetite.	Any fever or pain, especially if abdominal.	Check for other symptoms.
Vomiting.	See above - after diarrhoea.	See above.

Signs of Disease	Causes	Treatment and Prevention
NERVOUS SIGNS		
Head tilt to left or right side with circling to the tilted side.	Middle ear infection due to a variety of possible bacterial infections.	Early treatment with approprate antibiotic. General nursing care.
Above symptoms with head pressing and salivation.	Meningitis eg. Listeriosis bacterial infection.	Early treatment with antibiotic. Check feed for possible source of infection.
Above symptoms followed by collapse and convulsions.	Consider salt poisoning ie. water deprivation.	Remove feed and make sure animal can drink small amount regularly. Make sure all livestock have access at all times to clean, fresh water.
Muscle tremors followed by stiffness, rigidity and convulsions.	Tetanus (lockjaw) due to infection into a small wound which may or may not be found.	Antibiotic, antitoxin and sedatives. Good hygiene to prevent. Can also use vaccine on problem farms.
PROLAPSES		
Rectum.	Common in heavy, pregnant sows.	Can be replaced with vet attention. Cull after pigs are weaned.
Rectum and or vagina.	Common in heavy, pregnant sows.	Can be replaced and repaired with vet attention. Cull after pigs are weaned.
Uterine prolapse after farrowing.	Prolonged straining after farrowing is finished.	Acute vet emergency. Very difficult to treat and animal may die or have to be euthanased on welfare grounds.
THIN SOW SYNDROME		
	Insufficient feed. Worms, eg. gut or stomach worms. Poor housing causing draughts and wet bedding.	Improve feed, treat animals with anthelmintic, improve insulation within quarters and stop draughts.
VICES		
Bullying and fighting.	Poor husbandry.	Ensure adequate feed and trough space. Individual feeders are a good idea. Allow access to plenty of straw if in yards. Find the chief culprit and isolate.
If outdoors - excessive digging.	Natural habit.	Can be curbed by fitting nose rings.
SUDDEN DEATH		
Without prior warning.	Anthrax. Infection by Bacillus anthracis (NB. disease is notifiable and infectious to people). Erysipelas. Acute bacterial infection. Swine Fever. Virus infection (NB. notifiable disease). Heart Failure. Old, heavy sows are more prone to die this way. Erysipelas may be a factor in damaging the heart valves.	All sudden deaths should be notified to the vet. Disinfection is very important in limiting outbreak. Rare. Cull sows before they get too old and fat.

DIAGNOSTIC GUIDE TO PIGLET AILMENTS AND TREATMENT		
Signs of Disease	Causes	Prevention and Treatment
HEAD AND FACE		
Discharge from eyes.	Dusty environment causing irritation to eye membranes.	Improve ventilation and change bedding.
	Conjunctivitis due to bacterial infection.	Antibiotic eye cream.
	Rhinitis either Inclusion Body Rhinitis (herpes virus) or Atrophic (various bacterial agents).	Antibacterial, injectable and oral as treatment and control. Vaccine available for Atrophic control. Improve ventilation and hygiene.
Eyes dull and lifeless.	Part of any general disease or hypoglycaemia.	Check for other symptoms and treat accordingly.
Blindness.	Congenital defect causing eye malformations.	Nothing can be done. Check breeding policy.
Membranes of eye pale or white.	Anaemia iron deficiency.	All young pigs need iron injection in the first few days of life or oral iron until they are weaned to avoid anaemia.
Eyes sunk into sockets.	Dehydration as the result of scouring.	Electrolytes as fluid replacement. Scour may require antibiotic if infection is present.
Nasal discharge with sneezing.	Dusty environment.	Improve ventilation. Get rid of dust.
	Atrophic or Inclusion Body Rhinitis (see above).	Antibiotics can be used to treat, but must be used early in life (from a few days old) to be successful. Vaccine available for Atrophic Rhinitis. Improve ventilation and hygiene.
Twisted nostril to left or right, sometimes with difficulty breathing.	Either type of Rhinitis (see above).	See above and remember to buy in pigs from Rhinitis free sources.
Short snout: apart from what you would expect from breed.	May be Rhinitis but more likely if only a few involved to be congenital malformation.	If congenital nothing can be done.
Domed head.	Hydrocephalus.	Euthanasia on welfare grounds.
Salivation with sores in mouth and on snout.	Bacterial infection following an injury or virus infection eg. Foot and Mouth disease or Swine Vesicular disease (NB. both notifiable diseases).	Antibiotic. Get vet to check as if suspected viral cause need to notify ASAP.
Scabs and sores around face and cheeks.	Facial eczema/bacterial infection due to piglets fighting for a place at the udder.	Antibiotic and clip youngsters' teeth.
Inability to suckle.	Cleft palate.	Euthanasia on welfare grounds.

Signs of Disease	Causes	Treatment and Prevention
EARS		
One or both ears swollen.	Common cause is haematoma (blood blister). Less likely is abscess.	Better to leave haematoma if possible but if causing distress lance and then isolate the piglet. Abscesses must be lanced and drained and the patient given an antibiotic.
Brown discharge from one or both ears with some irritation.	Mange due to Sarcoptes scabiei. Unlikely in very young pigs.	Topical ectoparasiticides or injectable Ivermectin.
SKIN		
Absence of skin over an area at birth.	Inherited condition.	No treatment. May have to change breeding programme.
Skin covered with crusty brown discharge, non-itchy.	Greasy Pig Disease, usually pigs over 3 weeks old. Staph. hyicus infection.	Early treatment with antibiotic. Clean and disinfect accommodation. Clip youngsters' teeth.
Skin with brown discharge on back around eyes and ears, itchy.	Mange due to mite Sarcoptes scabiei.	Topical (eg. Porect) or injectable (Ivermectin) ectoparasiticides. Treat sows before farrowing and move to clean accommodation. Eradicate by treating all pigs every 10 days.
Skin itching without discharge.	Check for lice. Haematopinus suis.	Topical or injectable ectoparasitcides (see above).
Skin with round raised areas of reddened skin.	Pityriasis Rosea, cause unknown. Ringworm (NB. infectious to humans).	Will self-cure. Topical antifungal agent eg.Natamycin.
Skin covered in small, red sores that turn scabby.	Pig Pox due to a virus.	None required, will self-cure.
Skin with red raised sores (diamond shaped) mainly along back.	Swine Erysipelas (chronic infection) NOT in piglets, usually seen for the first time in fatteners.	Penicillin vaccine is highly effective.
Skin with blood blotches just under the skin in piglets just a few days old.	Haemolytic disease of the newborn, piglets often found dead.	Transfer remaining litter to other sow in milk or use milk substitute. Change the boar if a regular problem, cull the sow.
Skin with generalised redness, especially the ears.	If pigs are outdoors this is sunburn.	Provide shade and mud wallows.
Skin thickening with grey discolouration, non-itchy.	Parakeratosis ie. zinc deficiency. Pigs usually 2-4 months old.	Zinc supplement in the diet.
Skin with purple discolouration of ears and belly.	Any septicaemia can cause these symptoms, but consider in particular Salmonella and Swine Fever (NB. Salmonella infectious to people, Swine Fever a notifiable disease).	Get vet ASAP. Will need to look for other symptoms to make a diagnosis before treatment.

Signs of Disease	Causes	Treatment and Prevention
BREATHING		
Rapid breathing.	Stress due to pain or overheating or exercise. Pneumonia due to virus, bacteria or lungworm.	Identify and remove source of stress. If hyperthermic, apply cold water. Antibiotic by injection or in feed or water. Anthelmintic for lungworm. Get vet to check environment as well as treat animal.
Shallow breathing.	Probably asleep or possibly in terminal stage of illness.	No action. Check for other symptoms.
Coughing.	Respiratory disease eg. Pneumonia. In young pigs consider Barker Syndrome due to recessive gene. Outdoor pigs consider lungworm.	See above. Check breeding programme. Anthelmintic either oral or injectable. Move to clean pasture.
TEMPERATURE (normal range is 101.5 - 102.5°F)		
Raised.	Often as the result of infection by bacteria or virus. Pigs are very susceptible to hyperthermia in hot weather. Pain and stress can often cause a mild fever.	Further investigation required before treatment with antibiotic. Apply cold water. Sedative may be useful. Identify source of stress. Analgesics for pain.
Lowered.	Check again, may be incorrect technique. Baby pigs are very susceptible to low environmental temperatures if not feeding properly. May be terminally ill.	Raise temperatures with artifical heat (80-90°F). If sow has no milk foster piglets or give milk substitute or glucose and fluids. Check for other symptoms.
Sweating.	Pigs do not appear to sweat.	If pigs are too hot they lose heat through the skin. They also pant and use any source of water and mud to cool off.
Shivering.	See above for lowered temperature.	Pigs shiver to raise body temperature and also huddle together for warmth.
DUNG		
Constipation.	Not common in young pigs, but may be a secondary to Bowel Oedema.	Liquid paraffin or epsom salts in drinking water or bran in the feed.
Scouring. Neonatal pigs.	Baterial infection eg. E. coli, Clostridium or Campylobacter species. Virus infection eg. T.G.E. or Rotavirus.	Antibiotic, electrolytes, good nursing care. Vaccine can be helpful. Hygiene very important. General nursing care and electrolytes.
Age 1-3 weeks.	As above with the addition of Coccidiosis.	Treat affected with coccidiostat plus electrolytes. Prevent with good hygiene and treating sows with coccidiostat in feed prior to farrowing.

Signs of Disease	Causes	Treatment and Prevention
DUNG CONTINUED		
Post weaning.	Bacterial infection eg. E. coli and Salmonella (NB. infectious to people). Viral infection eg. T.G.E., Epidemic Diarrhoea. Worms eg. Ascaris or more likely Strongyloides, Oesophagostomum or Trichuris.	Antibiotic in feed or in drinking water. Good nursing care and electrolytes. Strict hygiene is essential and avoid stress. Anthelmintic and dose sows before farrowing to prevent infection in the litter.
Scouring with blood in the diarrhoea. Neonatal pigs.	Clostridial infection. Diarrhoea is often white with blood splashes. Campylobacter enteritis (Vibrio).	Antibiotic can help but antisera may be more useful. Vaccinate sows to protect the piglets. Antibiotic eg. Tylosin and Tiamutin may be most effective.
Age 1-3 weeks.	See above plus Coccidiosis.	As with all other types of scour with blood, vet needs to make diagnosis before treatment begins.
Post weaning.	As above for younger pigs, plus Swine Dysentery due to a spirochaete infection. Porcine Intestinal Adenomatosis (PIA) due to Campylobacter infection.	Lincocin, Tiamutin and Dimetridazole are drugs of choice in treatment. Good hygiene is essential. Tylosin is often drug of choice.
Vomiting.	Young pigs, Vomiting and Wasting disease due to Coronavirus. Other infections eg. T.G.E. can cause vomiting. but usually with diarrhoea.	No treatment. Try and expose sows and gilts to infection before farrowing. Check diagnosis.
Abdominal distention.	Gradual swelling of abdomen due to imperforate anus. Peritonitis - rare. Intestinal torsion.	Surgery rarely effective. Euthanase on welfare grounds. Do not breed from that sow again. Treatment unlikely to be effective. Pigs, usually weaners and older, commonly found dead or dying.
LAMENESS		
Feet.	Foot lesions in suckling pigs due mostly to poor flooring. Can lead to septic joints in the foot. Foot rot is a bacterial infection following damage to the foot. Foot and Mouth disease and Swine Vesicular disease (NB. both are notifiable diseases).Both are rare in UK.	Antibiotic can help, but improve the flooring. Early treatment with antibiotic. Contact your vet ASAP if suspicious.

Signs of Disease	Causes	Treatment and Prevention
LAMENESS CONTINUED		
Limbs.	Injury eg. fracture, nerve damage, puncture wounds and strain.	All but most minor will need some vet attention.
	Joint Ill ie. infection in the joints.	Antibiotic as soon as possible.
	Arthritis in fattening pigs due to Mycoplasma infection.	Antibiotic as soon as possible. (Lincocin often drug of choice).
	Splay leg congenital defect.	Do not breed affected pigs. Attention to flooring.
	Deficiency Disease eg. Osteomalacia/Rickets due to calcium/vitamin D deficiency.	Calcium and vitamin D supplements. Check diet for calcium phosphorus and vitamin D ratios.
	Osteochondrosis and Osteoarthritis due to rapid early growth.	Steroids/aspirin may help. Nursing and soft bedding.
Hind leg paralysis.	Injury.	Pain killers and soft bedding. If no response within a few days euthanase on welfare grounds.
	Spinal abscess often after tail biting.	No treatment.
BEHAVIOUR		
Loss of appetite.	Any fever or pain, especially if abdominal.	Check for other symptoms.
	Hypoglycaemia in youngsters due to lack of milk.	Fluids, glucose and warmth.
NERVOUS SIGNS		
Mild tremors when standing, gone when asleep.	Congenital tremors, six types recognised. Some due to congenital disorders, some due to virus infection.	Need further investigation. If due to virus may be Swine Fever (NB. a notifiable disease). If not may require changes to breeding programme.
Convulsions after head pressing and circling.	Salt poisoning or water deprivation.	Remove feed and allow controlled access to water. Ensure access to clean water at all times.
Uncoordination and loss of balance, squeaky voice, puffy eye lids, lateral recumbency and paddling of feet.	Bowel Oedema as the result of an Enterotoxaemia from E. coli.	Antibiotic corticosteroid. Avoid stress at weaning time and do not over feed at weaning.
Uncoordination and convulsions with high temperature.	Streptococcal Meningitis. Common in weaned pigs.	Antibiotic eg. ampicillin or penicillin most useful for treatment. In feed or in water antibiotic useful as prevention.
Muscle stiffness, stiff gait followed by convulsions.	Tetanus due to infection by Clostridium tetani into a wound.	Antibiotic, antisera and sedation. Good hygiene to prevent. Can also use vaccine on problem farms.

Signs of Disease	Causes	Treatment and Prevention
BEHAVIOUR CONTINUED		
VICES		
Tail, ear and flank biting.	Poor husbandry.	Ensure adequate feed and trough space. Check ventilation. Allow access to plenty of straw. Find the chief culprit and isolate and reduce stocking density.
BLEEDING DISORDERS		
Bleeding from navel.	Unknown. Occurs shortly after birth.	Ligate or clamp navel at birth. Vitamin K injections or supplements may be helpful.
Signs of bleeding in the skin and throughout the body.	Haemolytic disease of the newborn (see above).	Transfer litters to other sows or use milk substitutes. Use different boar if a herd problem. Cull the sow.
SUDDEN DEATH		
Without prior warning.	Anthrax ie. infection by Bacillus anthracis (NB. a notifiable disease when animal is dead and infectious to people).	All sudden deaths must be notified to vet. Vaccine available. Disinfection is very important in limiting outbreak.
	Swine Erysipelas. Bacterial infection.	Vaccine available.
	Swine Fever (NB. a notifiable disease). Virus infection.	Rare in UK.
	Stress syndrome. Stress precipitates onset in pigs with genetic defect.	Avoid stressing pigs at all times eg. do not feed fat pigs prior to leading. Breed out defect.
	Slurry poisoning. Gases given off by slurry without adequate ventilation can be poisonous.	Care required on investigation. Improve ventilation.
	Electrocution. Faulty wiring.	Extreme care required on investigation. Get qualified person to check wiring etc.

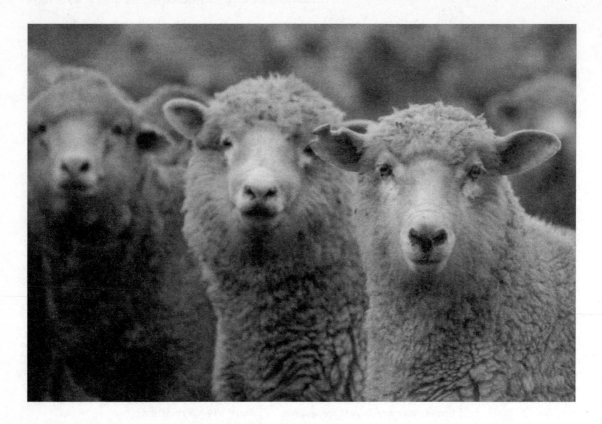

Chapter Six

SOME COMMON DISEASES AFFECTING SHEEP

By Jane Upton and Denis Soden

It is always alarming to read about the numerous diseases to which sheep, like any other animal, can succumb, but good management, sensible fencing, anticipation of potential troubles and quick reaction will ensure that disasters rarely happen.

Blowfly Strike

This is probably the most common and troublesome of all diseases during the warmer months from April to November. The green or blue blowfies, which are slightly larger than houseflies, actively seek sites where they can lay their eggs and where the hatching maggots can obtain food. The fly finds the sheep particularly attractive when there are faeces contaminating the tail area, but even without this the natural smell of the sheep is sufficient to entice the fly to lay its eggs on the wool, and any open wounds can suffer the same fate. The eggs hatch in a few hours and the maggots start feeding by burrowing into the skin. The debris they create attracts more flies, and within a very short time the area affected rapidly increases in size.

However, long before this happens, the behaviour of the sheep will indicate to the observant shepherd that it requires attention. Sheep which have newly hatched maggots will be irritated by them and will waggle their tails vigorously. They may stamp the ground with a hind foot and twist the whole body from side to side while holding the head high in the air. The sheep must be caught and examined carefully. Apply a combined insecticide and antiseptic to the site of the maggots and also the surrounding wool to catch any that attempt to escape, rubbing the medication into the fleece with the fingertips.

If the strike is left untreated, the next indication will be a dark stain on the surface of the wool which is caused by the excreta from the maggots. By now the sheep will be feeling very sick and may be lying by itself under a tree or hedge. If moved it will stand with its head lowered and quickly lie down again.

In July and August the blowfly often lays eggs on the back of the sheep near the shoulders. When the maggots develop there, the sheep will stand with its head lowered and appear to be very sick. The tail waggling and body twisting are absent and one of the few visual signs is the tell-tale dark stain starting on the back and running down on to the shoulders. This appears after the maggots have been feeding for a day or two. Try to recognise the situation and deal with it before this.

Any sheep which have footrot are also at risk, as the distinctive smell of footrot attracts the blowfly to lay its eggs, and the resulting maggots penetrate the under-run hoof. Trim off the under-run sole and saturate with an insecticidal and antiseptic dressing.

Adult sheep are at risk of fly strike from late April until they are shorn. They are then free from infection until the wool has grown to around 20cm, after which they can be protected for a few weeks by using a pour-on preparation such as Vetrazin. Lambs, unless they are shorn, are at risk all through the summer, but they too can be protected by using a pour-on preparation.

Blowfly strike is less likely to occur if preventative measures are taken routinely. Wool contaminated after lambing or as a consequence of diarrhoea should be cut off. Shearing is usually carried out in June but in exceptionally mild weather in the south of England it can be brought forward to the end of April. Clean, freshly shorn sheep are unlikely to suffer.

Sheep Scab

Sheep scab is caused by a mite which burrows into the skin and causes intense itching, along with rapid loss of wool and condition, and it requires immediate attention. If an infection is suspected, contact the vet immediately. He will be able to suggest the most effective treatment.

Scab is contagious and will rapidly spread through the flock if untreated. It is still a notifiable disease and unfortunately has become much more prevalent since annual dipping of sheep ceased to be compulsory. The disease will get into the flock only if there is very close contact with infected sheep or recently contaminated equipment, so it is wise to isolate, and if necessary treat, all sheep brought in before allowing them to mix with the flock.

Orf

Orf (Contagious Pustular Dermatitis) is a very

painful condition affecting sheep of all ages. It is caused by a virus which enters the skin through minor cuts and abrasions, and it can also affect humans who come into contact with infected sheep, causing painful, scabby areas on the hands, wrists, inner arms and face. For this reason it is necessary to wear protective gloves at all times when dealing with this disease.

Having penetrated the skin, the virus multiplies rapidly, causing small spots which suppurate and join together to form grape-like clusters. It is confined to the non-woolly areas in both ewes and lambs. In lactating ewes the udders and teats become infected, and in young lambs it affects the lips, gums and nose, resulting in the doubly distressing situation where hungry lambs with painful mouths are prevented from feeding because of the soreness and pain in the ewes' teats. The condition clears up in a few weeks and healing occurs. Orf can also affect older weaned lambs in the autumn and the genital areas of ewes and rams, making the rams very reluctant to work. The condition known as strawberry footrot which causes raw red bleeding areas on the non-woolly areas of the faces and legs is believed to be related to the orf virus.

Being a virus, orf does not respond to antibiotics and is virtually impossible to cure. Secondary infections of the lesions can be guarded against by the use of an antibiotic spray.

It is possible to vaccinate against orf. The vaccine is applied to an area of bare skin, preferably between a foreleg and the chest wall. Do not use disinfectant or spirit to clean the skin before applying the vaccine, which is a modified form of the living virus, as this would destroy it before it can produce the desired effect. The skin must be lightly scratched where the vaccine is applied, and later a scab will form.

The disease is most troublesome in lactating ewes with newborn lambs, and flocks in which orf has occurred previously should be vaccinated two months before protection is required. On no account should sheep in flocks where the disease has never occurred be vaccinated. This is because the mild infection introduced by the modified living virus produces scabs at the site of the vaccination and these, as they fall from the sheep, are liable to affect any 'clean' sheep bought in.

An outbreak of orf can be controlled to a certain extent, especially in young suckling lambs, by vaccinating non-affected members of the flock. Seek the advice of your vet if an outbreak occurs, and follow the manufacturer's instructions carefully when using the vaccine.

Lameness

Lameness can occur in a number of different ways. Watch the sheep to see how it moves and which is the lame leg or legs. Catch the sheep, immobilise it and examine each foot in turn.

One of the commonest forms of lameness is caused by vegetable matter and mud becoming impacted between the hooves, and by mud becoming trapped in the layer of horn on the hoof wall of overgrown feet. Once this is removed and the hoof pared, the sheep will quickly become sound.

Look for a reddened and moist area between the digits and also for abscesses around the top of the hoof. If these are not found, feel the leg for any hot spots or swelling which might indicate a sprain or hairline fracture. Check that there are no dislocated joints.

Footrot and Scald

Footrot is a very painful and debilitating disease if allowed to go untreated and is directly responsible for causing huge financial losses to the sheep industry every year. While it is not a killer disease in itself, it can severely affect the performance of all classes of sheep, from young lambs and ewes to rams, the latter especially at mating time.

It is caused by the joint action of several types of organisms, one of which is quite common in some areas of the UK. It causes scald – an inflammation of the skin between the two digits of the foot – and it can occur in all classes of sheep at any time of the year, but is more commonly seen when the sheep, particularly lambs, are grazing long, lush grass in the spring, and also shortly after ewes have been housed on straw bedding in the winter. The particular organism which causes scald can only live for three weeks away from the sheep, and careful use of a footbath can eradicate it from the flock, especially if clean land is available for grazing after footbathing.

True footrot occurs when a second organism invades the inflamed tissue between the digits. This causes an under-running of the sole of the foot, and eventually the horny outer wall, reaching right up to the toe. If this under-run tissue is lifted or pared off, the exposed area resembles the gills of a mushroom, except that it is usually dark grey in colour, and has a characteristic pungent, unpleasant smell. Treatment consists of paring away all the under-run horn from the sole and outer surface of the digit. The bulk of the material can be cut away with straight-bladed secateurs, but a very sharp knife should be used for the more precise trimming necessary to expose the fullest extent of the infection. The dividing line between healthy and infected tissue is a very fine one, and every care should be taken to avoid the bleeding which will occur if the healthy tissue is cut, especially in the region of the toe.

Here it should be stated that if footrot is treated as soon as a sheep is seen to be walking lame, a lot of pain for the sheep and a lot of work for the shepherd can be avoided. An antibiotic spray can be used to treat the infection, and the sheep should be stood on a hard surface while the foot dries.

When footrot or scald is present, it is much easier to control if all the sheep can be stood in a shallow bath of 10 percent zinc sulphate solution for up to an hour. This long period enables the solution to penetrate pockets where the causal organisms might have been missed when paring. The feet should then be allowed to dry before returning to pasture. Formalin is also used for treatment and control, but it has a number of disadvantages. The fumes given off are toxic, and it is ineffective when the footbath becomes contaminated with dung or soil. It makes the hoof very hard and is very painful if used on feet where footrot has already been exposed. The feet should be soaked for a much shorter time with formalin solution, about two minutes usually being sufficient.

Both zinc sulphate and formalin are difficult to dispose of and both are poisonous to fish if allowed into streams, ponds or ditches. Zinc sulphate may be used and reused as it does not deteriorate in contact with vegetable matter.

When treating footrot it is important that all foot parings are collected and burnt and that all tools are disinfected by immersing them in 10 prcent zinc sulphate solution between each sheep.

In severe cases of footrot, and particularly with valuable rams, consult a veterinary surgeon about the possibility of an antibiotic injection as treatment after paring. Prevention can be assisted by using a footrot vaccine. Two vaccinations are required initially, followed by two booster injections each year. The vaccine is expensive to buy and any partly used bottles must be discarded, which adds to the expense for small flock owners.

Foot Abscesses

These can cause very painful lameness, occurring where the horn of the hoof joins the skin of the coronet. Consult your veterinary surgeon.

Granulomas or Proudflesh

When the feet are allowed to become badly overgrown, the horn may aggravate the soft tissue between the digits, or the under-run sole may rub against the sensitive layer below it and cause excessive growth with associated bleeding, especially from the area of the toe. This is a very painful condition and in the spring and summer may attract the blowfly to lay its eggs in the foot. (This is also the case with ordinary footrot).

Granulomas need to be surgically removed by a vet and even so they take a long time to heal.

Roundworms

All sheep carry some worms but it is the balance between numbers and the state of the sheep's resistance which determines whether disease develops. Pasture management is an important factor in controlling roundworm population. The old saying 'A sheep's worst enemy is another sheep' indicates that heavy stocking rates, coupled with infrequent moves onto clean pasture, can result in heavy infestation, with a resultant loss in condition and a reduced growth rate.

Roundworms occur in a variety of forms. Those that cause problems for sheep start life as eggs passed out with the faeces onto the pasture. Given suitable climatic conditions of warmth and moisture, the eggs develop into larvae which go through several stages before migrating onto grass stems where they are eaten by sheep. Two weeks later they are mature adults, mating and producing eggs.

This is an oversimplification of the matter because different types of roundworm prefer different parts of the digestive tract in which to live and produce eggs. Some can lie dormant in the gut until favourable conditions for further development come along. When this happens, a rapid explosion of activity occurs. Some types hibernate through the winter as larval stages on the pasture and only when the temperature rises in the spring (which also stimulates the growth of new grass) do they hatch in massive numbers to be eaten by young lambs and cause a lot of problems.

Diarrhoea, dehydration and reduced appetite are symptoms which can indicate worm infestation, although these can be confused with symptoms of other conditions. Even with moderate or light infestations there will be a reduced growth rate in the lambs and the fleeces will appear dull, dry and lacking in bloom.

Anthelmintics are drugs that control internal parasites and a wide range of them is available for the control of roundworms. For the treatment to be effective, it is very important to follow the manufacturer's instructions carefully to match the dosage required to the weight of the animal being treated. There is evidence that some types of roundworm are becoming resistant to some of the drugs being used. Check with your vet as to the most suitable anthelmintic if your sheep have a particular problem.

Clean pasture is invaluable in providing an efficient management aid in that newly dosed sheep can graze without the challenge of immediate re-infestation. Similarly, mixed grazing with cattle can do a lot to reduce the uptake of worm larvae.

Tapeworms

Tapeworms are flat, ribbon-like parasites which live in the small intestine of the sheep. The worm consists of a tiny head which attaches itself to the wall of the gut, either by a sucker or with hooks, and it feeds in that position. The ribbon-like body consists of a series of segments which are grown from the head and which may reach several metres in length. They are in fact packets of eggs which are shed from the end of the worm and pass out with the faeces. They require an intermediate host for their further development, and can be easily seen as flat, white, short pieces of tape. Although unsightly, they rarely cause any great harm to the sheep, unless present in large numbers.

Many anthelmintics used to control roundworms are also effective with tapeworms. Details will be found on the manufacturer's package.

Gid

There are a number of different kinds of tapeworm, and this disease of the central nervous system is caused when sheep eat grass contaminated by the larval stage of a tapeworm found in dogs. Over a period of time the larvae migrate through the bloodstream and begin developing when they reach the nervous tissue, including the brain. Here they grow into a cyst filled with fluid containing tapeworm heads.

The symptoms which may indicate gid can vary, and are easily confused with other nervous diseases. Sometimes the affected sheep will lie with the head turned to one side, or hold it abnormally high. Others will walk in circles, always turning the same way, and all will eventually go down, become comatose and die. The time taken for this to happen varies considerably, and if the veterinary surgeon is called in early and diagnoses gid, the chances are that he will be able to operate successfully and remove the cyst.

If the uncooked head of a dead sheep suffering from gid is eaten by a dog, the tapeworm heads develop into adult tapeworms and the life cycle of the parasite begins again. It is possible to break this cycle by ensuring that any sheep offal fed to dogs is boiled for at least one hour. All dogs owned should be dosed with a medication obtainable from your vet, which is capable of killing all of these tapeworms, including the heads. This should be done every two months, but of course it will not prevent other dogs and foxes coming onto the property and contaminating the grassland.

Hydatid Disease

There is another type of tapeworm, less than a centimetre in length, which lives in the small intestine of dogs. The ripe segments from these tiny tapeworms are passed out in the faeces of the dog, some adhering to the hairy coat. Infection of the sheep occurs when the grazing animal eats grass contaminated by infected dogs. Humans, especially children, can become infected by stroking and cuddling dogs and then accidentally swallowing the tapeworm eggs.

The hydatid cyst will grow in any part of the body, but commonly in the lungs and liver. Human beings cannot become infected by eating lamb or mutton. Prevention is by strict hygiene when handling dogs and by dosing them regularly with an anthelmintic against this particular tapeworm, called Echinococcus granulosus. Never feed raw sheep meat to dogs – it should be cooked for at least an hour – and dispose of any carcases so that they cannot be scavenged by dogs or foxes. Discuss prevention with your vet.

Liver Fluke

The fluke is a flat, leaf-like parasite which is common in wet, marshy areas. It requires an intermediate host, a mud snail, for its development. For the sheep, the problem starts when it eats grass which is carrying the encysted stage of the fluke. On reaching the sheep's gut, the immature fluke makes its way through the gut wall and searches out the liver. Once in the liver it feeds voraciously, and on becoming adult it anchors itself in the bile duct and takes blood from the wall. It lays eggs which pass out with the faeces. These then hatch and seek out a mud snail, in which they multiply, thereafter leaving the snail and encysting themselves on grass to begin the cycle again.

Affected sheep become very anaemic and lose condition. A watery swelling appears under the lower jaw and the membranes of the eyes and mouth become very pale.

If the presence of fluke is suspected, take a dung sample to your vet who will be able to tell you whether fluke eggs are present. The vet will also advise on the method of treatment most pertinent to the condition of your sheep. Cattle, goats, deer and rabbits can also act as hosts and carriers of fluke.

Pulpy Kidney and Other Causes of Sudden Death

There is a group of diseases (including tetanus) caused by Clostridium bacteria which can cause sudden death, and it is very nearly always the best sheep which are affected. Fortunately there are very good vaccines available which will give complete protection from specific diseases if given routinely and according to the manufacturer's instructions. It is recommended that for all breeding stock a '7 in 1' type vaccine is used. If well grown and sold for slaughter before 16 weeks of age, lambs born in a vaccinated flock will not normally need vaccination, as the protection given by antibodies in the ewe's colostrum will be sufficient. Other vaccines giving protection against fewer clostridial diseases are available.

It should always be assumed that any bought-in sheep are unvaccinated. They should be given a full dose of vaccine immediately, followed by a booster dose four weeks later. Another booster dose for the ewes four weeks before lambing commences ensures that newborn lambs are protected, provided they get an adequate supply of colostrum. If lambing is protracted it may be necessary to give a further booster dose of vaccine to late-lambing ewes.

Home-bred ewe lambs born to vaccinated ewes and intended as flock replacements will require a primary vaccination at two to three months of age, followed by a secondary dose four to six weeks later. If they are bred from in their first year they, like the ewes, will require a booster dose four weeks before lambing. Similarly, ram lambs kept for breeding should be treated like the ewe lambs, but in subsequent years a booster dose around four weeks before mating commences will suffice.

This vaccine should be given subcutaneously at a site high on the neck of the sheep. Occasionally an abscess or nodule may form at the injection site. If this is on the neck it will not reduce the value of the skin after slaughter.

Pneumonia

The bacteria which cause pneumonia in sheep come in many different types. Deaths from pneumonia can occur in all classes of sheep and at any time of the year. Often the first sign of the disease is a dead sheep, or a short period of laboured breathing and frothing at the mouth followed by death. Other forms of the disease can be treated with long-acting antibiotics if detected early.

Pasteurellosis (pneumonia)

This is a very complex and variable condition. Periods of stress, which can include bad weather, can predispose a flock to infection, and if the level of stress is great enough outbreaks can occur even though the sheep have been vaccinated.

A post-mortem examination of sheep which die from pneumonia will reveal plum-coloured lungs surrounded by bloodstained fluid, and in many cases death occurs so rapidly that it is impossible to observe any symptoms.

It is possible to vaccinate against certain types of pasteurella, and to be effective the vaccine must be appropriate to the particular requirements of the flock as determined by laboratory tests. It is possible to buy a combined clostridial and pasteurella vaccine, but little, if any, immunity to pasteurella is passed to the lambs in the antibodies contained in the colostrum, compared to the cover given against the clostridial diseases. If early protection is required for the lambs they must be given pasteurella-only vaccine when two weeks old if they are born to ewes which have previously been vaccinated.

Lambs born to ewes which have not been vaccinated can be given pasteurella-only vaccine

at birth, followed two weeks later by a second injection. Ewe lambs retained for breeding will require one annual booster injection.

Metabolic Diseases

Metabolic diseases associated with feeding and production are sudden in onset and can lead to death in a very short time. They arise as a consequence of food intake not meeting urgent requirements.

Pregnancy Toxaemia

Also known as twin lamb disease, this occurs during the last month of pregnancy, most commonly in ewes that are carrying two or three lambs. At this time the unborn lambs are making heavy nutritional demands on the ewe. Pregnancy toxaemia can affect both thin and fat ewes and is usually caused by an insufficient uptake of nutritious food.

Concentrates should be fed during the last six weeks of pregnancy, starting with 100g per day, increasing weekly to reach 750g per day by lambing. The protein content of the concentrates should be 17 percent, and it is helpful if the merchant supplying the feed gives you a list of the ingredients so that the stated analysis can be checked.

Ewes affected by pregnancy toxaemia get separated from the rest of the flock, refuse food and become blind. After a few days they are unable to stand and they assume unnatural positional behaviour. Front legs may be stretched out in front and the head pressed down into the ground. Symptoms include twitching and trembling of the lips and ears, and grinding teeth. If the ewe is left untreated, death follows fairly quickly. The advice of the vet should be quickly sought if pregnancy toxaemia is suspected, and the ewe moved to warm, comfortable conditions under cover.

Prevention of this disease is easier if sheep are housed, as a more careful check can be kept on their condition. The target condition score at lambing is 3.5 (loin full, moderate fat cover), and thin ewes and shy feeders which are often bullied at the trough should be separated and given extra concentrates. Ewes which are lame or have teeth problems are also at risk, as are ewes kept outside in periods of very bad weather. See that all the ewes have sufficient trough space and put all the feed in the troughs before allowing the sheep access to it, perhaps in a separate enclosure or an adjoining field. This will allow fair shares for all.

The bulk of the diet should be good quality hay with the concentrate fed first. A stomach full of poor quality food is of no use to a ewe carrying three lambs. Four-fifths of the eventual birthweight is gained during the last two months of pregnancy.

Overfat ewes too are at risk, simply because internal layers of fat restrict the space available for any increase in nutritious food required to feed the unborn lambs.

Death is caused by a breakdown of the metabolism and a lowering of blood sugar levels. One school of thought suggests that if the ewe is shorn the metabolism is stirred into action again by the demands of the ewe as she attempts to convert energy into warmth!

It is best to prevent the disease by careful management of the flock, particularly in the later stages of pregnancy, as the recovery rate is very low.

Hypocalcaemia

This disease can occur during late pregnancy or early lactation, and it is caused by a low level of calcium in the blood. Listlessness and depression precede loss of consciousness, but a subcutaneous injection of 100ml of 20 percent calcium borogluconate will effect a rapid return to normal. Divide the dose and inject at five or six different sites on the body.

Hypomagnesaemia

The onset of this disease can be extremely rapid and usually occurs when newly lambed ewes are turned out onto very lush grass. It is caused by low levels of magnesium in the blood, and is characterised by a stiffness when walking, and twitching and spasms, followed by convulsions and death. Prompt treatment consisting of a subcutaneous injection of 100ml of magnesium fortified with 20 percent calcium borogluconate divided and injected at several sites as with hypocalcaemia, is necessary.

The main problem in treating this disease is the speed at which it develops, and unless the person in charge is present and very observant, quite often the only indication is a dead sheep. Prevention can be assisted by offering a mineral mixture containing calcined magnesite, but as this is an unpalatable ingredient it needs to be disguised to make it acceptable by adding some molasses or treacle. It is possible to buy compound feeds containing calcined magnesite, and these should be introduced into the rations gradually just before lambing, and continued for a few weeks afterwards while animals are at risk.

Heavy dressings of nitrogenous fertilisers encourage a rapid growth of young grass in the spring which also reduces the uptake of both calcium and magnesium, a point to be borne in mind when considering how best to manage the available grassland.

Diseases Associated with Lambing

Abortion

There are a number of different organisms which can cause abortion in sheep. Abortion can also be caused by other factors such as worrying dogs, malnutrition, incorrect handling and being forced too quickly through narrow gateways, to name but a few. In some cases of abortion early or midway through pregnancy the foetus may be so small that it passes unnoticed by the shepherd. A single ewe aborting may give no cause for alarm and be dismissed as one of the accepted risks of keeping livestock.

When a number of abortions occur, producing dead or very weakly foetuses, the vet should be called in without delay as it is only by microscopic bacteriological examination of aborted material that an accurate diagnosis can be made, and, if appropriate, the type of vaccine required to minimise further losses be recommended.

Domestic cats are responsible for spreading infection causing one type of abortion in sheep, which is also contagious to humans. Consequently, extreme care should be taken when handling and disposing of any aborted material, and pregnant women should stay away from ewes at lambing time.

Mastitis

Mastitis can be present in the ewe flock in both chronic and acute forms. The chronic form is usually discovered when the ewes are being inspected prior to selection for the breeding flock. It is identifiable as a fibrous lump or series of lumps in the udder. If the ewe is used for breeding, the affected side of the udder will not produce any milk. It is not

known when infection occurs and there is no known cure. Affected ewes should be culled.

The acute form commonly occurs early in lactation. Affected ewes are clearly ill and appear to be walking stiffly, and the udder is swollen and grows increasingly cold to the touch. The udder rapidly becomes inflamed, turning red or purplish-blue and eventually black. If the teat is drawn, a bloodstained fluid comes away. The inflammation may extend along the belly of the ewe if she survives and eventually all the dead coloured tissue will fall off, leaving a raw, bleeding surface. Healing takes a long time and the exposed tissue is vulnerable to fly strike. Consult the vet as to the best course of action. There is no effective treatment for this condition and if the ewe survives she should be culled.

Navel Infections

The umbilical cord of a newborn lamb is moist and immediately after birth it is in contact with many different types of bacteria on the ground. This is the route by which certain harmful organisms gain entry to the body of the lamb. It is comparatively easy to prevent this from happening by applying an antiseptic dressing to the navel as soon as the lamb is born and then placing the lamb on a bed of clean straw. The aim is to dry up the cord as quickly as possible and to disinfect the area of the body around it.

Several preparations are suitable for use as a dressing:
• Tincture of iodine
• Antibiotic aerosol
• A weak solution of copper sulphate
A dressing which can be contained in a wide-necked bottle is actually preferable to an aerosol as the wet cord and the area immediately surrounding it can be totally immersed in the

liquid. Hold the lamb vertically by its forelegs and put the navel cord into the neck of the bottle. Lift the bottle at a right angle to the lamb and press it gently into the belly.

Coccidiosis

Coccidiosis is a disease of young lambs. Any older sheep will have developed an immunity through previous contact with the parasite, but they can still pass on the infection. The disease occurs mostly in housed flocks, although it can also infect lambs on heavily stocked pasture through contaminated faeces.

Infected lambs become unthrifty with a loss of appetite and develop a mild diarrhoea which causes dehydration. If coccidiosis is suspected, consult your vet over treatment and preventative measures to be taken in subsequent years.

Notifiable Diseases

Notifiable diseases include bluetongue, foot and mouth disease, anthrax, brucellosis (and Johne's disease in Northern Ireland). I have not dealt with them in detail because they are thankfully still rare, although I have included bluetongue because there are steps which the responsible sheep keeper can take to limit the spread of this disease. For further information please refer to the diagnostic tables.

Bluetongue

The most recent concern for the sheep keeping community is bluetongue. It is spread by the cullicoides midge and arrived in the UK in 2007, although at the time the onset of winter limited its effects. Due to its primary method of transmission the government opted for a programme of vaccination which is mandatory only in Scotland, but strongly recommended

by all the relevant organisations across the UK. Prime risk periods are from mid-summer to early autumn and it is recommended that the whole flock is vaccinated, with the exception of lambs less than one month old. Full immunity occurs three months after vaccination.

Inspect stock regularly with particular emphasis on the lining of the mouth and nose and the point at which the hoof ends and skin begins (known as the coronary band). Symptoms include eye and nasal discharges, drooling, high body temperature, swelling in the mouth, head and neck, lameness and wasting of muscles in the hind legs, respiratory problems, fever, lethargy, inflammation of the coronary band and haemorrages either into or under the skin.

At present there are uncertainties regarding the spread of bluetongue with a belief that transmission can also occur by mechanical means from flock to flock or by unhygienic practices with items such as syringes. What is certain is the the seriousness of bluetongue, which is a notifiable disease. Any suspicion of its presence must be reported immediately to your local Animal Health Office, details of which are available from Defra's helpline on 08459 335577.

Zoonoses

Animal diseases which are communicable to human beings are called zoonoses, and while some may cause only slight problems, others can be dangerous and even life-threatening. Anyone who is working with sheep or in contact with them when a zoonotic disease is present or suspected should seek medical advice without delay if they feel unwell.

Zoonotic diseases include anthrax, rabies, samonellosis, hydatid disease, orf, brucellosis, chlamydiosis, listeriosis, toxoplasmosis and all abortion agents. The last five on this list all pose a threat to pregnant women as they can cause abortion or serious defects if in contact with the unborn foetus. Pregnant women should keep away from sheep at lambing time.

Some Plants Poisonous To Sheep

Most poisonous plants are avoided by sheep unless grazing is very sparse as in times of drought or during spells of severe weather, especially snowstorms. The main danger comes when they are cut, wilted and made into hay, often unnoticed, and are then readily eaten by the sheep.

▪ Yew is probably the plant which causes most problems for the small flock owner. If only a small quantity is eaten the animal will die. This applies to the living shrub or the tree, and also to any hedge trimmings which may inadvertently be dumped where the sheep have access to them.

▪ Bracken is poisonous to stock but to a much lesser extent than yew, and will normally be eaten only when grazing is in short supply or when it is made into hay or used as bedding. Sheep affected by bracken poisoning become blind.

▪ Equisetum or horsetail is not usually a problem unless cut, dried and made into hay. If it is then eaten it is poisonous and there is no antidote. The sheep will die.

▪ Laburnum seems to affect sheep less than some other types of livestock when eaten. All parts of the tree are poisonous and will cause death if consumed in quantity.

▪ Acorns are sometimes eaten in quantity by sheep who inexplicably develop a craving for them. They are more poisonous when green and unripe. Affected animals suffer from constipation, which is then quickly followed by

diarrhoea. They should be moved away from the source as quickly as possible.

▪ Azaleas and rhododendrons often 'escape' into boundary fences from gardens and woodlands and can cause considerable damage to the nervous system if eaten. As with yew, the clippings from gardens are as toxic when wilted as when green. The shrub should either be removed completely or fenced off out of reach of the sheep, as ewes seeking extra nutrition in the weeks just prior to lambing will readily eat it, having avoided it completely for months before.

▪ Ragwort. This should be pulled out and burned before it reaches the flowering stage. The toxin accumulates in sheep if they are given hay containing the dried plant.

Your Veterinary Surgeon

Some veterinary surgeons are more involved with sheep than others, so try to find and get to know one with whom you can readily communicate. Also, do this before you encounter an emergency. It will cost you money, but a general advisory visit to discuss management, feeding, a vaccination programme, a worming policy, etc., could prove to be a very good investment.

Don't forget that you can also take a sheep which is in trouble to the surgery and save yourself a call-out fee!

DIAGNOSTIC GUIDE TO SHEEP AILMENTS AND TREATMENT

Signs of Disease	Causes	Treatment and Prevention
HEAD AND FACE		
Nasal discharge.	Pneumonia due to virus or bacterial infection. Most common infection is due to Pasteurella. Watery discharge from nostrils may be due to Jaagsiekte (Pulmonary Adenomatosis).	Antibiotic for most cases. If indoors check ventilation. A vaccine is available for preventon of Pasteurella. No treatment. No vaccine available.
Nasal discharge with pus and blood.	Sheep nasal fly. Seen only in the summer months.	Ivermectin may be useful as can organophosphorus dips and pour on insecticides.
Ulcers on lips, tongue and dental pad.	Foot and Mouth disease (NB. notifiable disease).	Check for other symptoms eg. blisters on feet. If suspicious inform vet and authorities.
Scabs around eyes, ears and base of horns.	Facial eczema or eye scab due to bacterial infection, Staph. aureus. Head fly. Photosensitisation may also be a factor in summer months.	Antibiotic, usually injectable. Isolate affected animals and increase trough space. Pour on insecticide. Eating St. John's wort or clover may precipitate condition. Move to other pasture or indoors. Treat with steroids or antihistamines.
Loss of hair on face, especially around the eyes.	Ringworm, usually due to Trychophyton verrucosum. Rare condition. (NB. infectious to people).	Topical antifungal agents.
Salivation and drooling from the mouth.	Virus infection (see Foot and Mouth above). Actinobacillosis ie. bacterial infection in the mouth, jaw bone and elsewhere. Foreign body stuck in mouth or throat. Might have tooth problems or abscess or tumour.	See Foot and Mouth. Antibiotic or sodium iodide intravenous weekly or potassium iodide orally daily. Abdomen may be blowing up with gas. Emergency situation. If unable to dislodge or push into stomach a trocar and cannula in rumen may be necessary to relieve bloat. Tumour - no treatment viable. Dental treatment may be an option.
Swelling of face and tongue.	Bluetongue or Foot & Mouth disease (NB. both notifiable diseases).	No effective treatment. Vaccinate for Bluetongue.
Fluid swelling under jaw.	Chronic fluke infection.	Routine treatment with fluke preparation used both as treatment and prevention. Drain land and try to get rid of the snail which is the intermediate host.
EYES		
Watery discharge from one or both eyes.	Entropion ie. inturned eye lid(s). Usually rectified as young animal.	Minor surgery required. See vet.
Swollen eye lids.	Allergic reaction.	Antihistamine or corticosteroid injections. May have to move pastures.

Signs of Disease	Causes	Treatment and Prevention
EYES CONTINUED		
White discharge from one or both eyes, sometimes with damage to the surface of the eye.	Infectious Kerato-conjunctivitis due to infection by Rickettsia or Chlamydia organism.	Subconjunctival injection (job for the vet) or topical antibiotic ointment. Control is difficult. Reduce crowding.
Discharge from one eye with or without eye damage.	Look for foreign body in the eye eg. hay seed.	Careful search and remove after putting local anaesthetic in eye. Will need antibiotic eye ointment.
Eyes dull and lifeless.	Part of any general disease condition eg. Toxaemia.	Look for other symptoms before beginning treatment. If in doubt get vet.
Blindness with obvious eye lesions.	Cataracts. Damage to surface after infection or trauma.	Nothing practical can be done. Topical antibiotic and steroid cream may be helpful.
Blindness with no obvious eye damage.	Rape or other brassica poisoning. Bracken poisoning. Any form of brain degeneration caused by infection eg. abscesses or Toxaemia eg. Pregnancy Toxaemia.	Remove from field. Remove from source. Antibiotic and thiamine may help. Check for other symptoms to make a full diagnosis before beginning treatment.
Yellow colour in the white of the eye.	Jaundice usually the result of copper poisoning or chronic liver disease eg. Fascioliasis.	Oral dose of sodium sulphate. Prognosis is poor. Treat with fluke remedies.
Membranes of the eye pale or white.	Anaemia due to worms or fluke. Deficiency disease eg. due to lack of copper, cobalt or iron in the diet.	Treat with anthelmintic. Copper or cobalt boluses but only after a definite diagnosis has been made by blood testing.
Membranes of the eye dark and congested.	Circulatory difficulties as part of a more general disease eg. Pneumonia.	Check for other symptoms. If in doubt see vet.
Eyes sunk into sockets.	Dehydration usually as the result of scouring.	Electrolyte and fluid therapy and treat the cause of the scour.
EARS		
One or both ears swollen.	Abscess or blood blister ie. haematoma.	Drain abscess and give antibiotic. If haematoma leave to reabsorb naturally.
One ear drooping with possible discharge from one ear canal.	Bacterial infection or possible Listeriosis.	Antibiotic. If Listeriosis consider source of infection eg. silage. Also practise good hygiene in lambing pen.
SKIN AND FLEECE		
Loss of fleece with scabs and itching.	Sheep scab due to Psoroptic mite infection. Any untreated sheep with infection may be welfare cases and owner prosecuted if left unattended.	Dip with approved sheep scab dip. Ensure all safety precautions are observed when dipping.
Severe itching with nervous symptoms.	Scrapie (NB. notifiable disease) due to infection by a small virus-like particle.	No treatment. All infected animals should be slaughtered.

Signs of Disease	Causes	Treatment and Prevention
SKIN AND FLEECE CONTINUED		
Loss of fleece with itching. Parasites found.	Lice, ticks and keds could all be involved.	Dip or spray or pour on affected animals with recommended products. This may have to be repeated every 10 - 14 days.
Wet staining of wool mostly around the rear end and with the animal distressed.	Blowfly maggots.	Dip or spray or pour on with recommended products affected and non-affected animals. Dag the flock ie. clean or clip the area of the dock. Severely affected animals may have to be put down.
Discolouration of the fleece with crusting of the wool. No distress to the animal.	Dermatophilus infection, often common in cool, wet weather.	Injectable antibiotic can be helpful. Keep animals dry. Alum dips may be helpful.
Wrinkled skin with sores.	Zinc deficiency. Rare condition.	Zinc sulphate weekly . Control with zinc fertiliser on pasture.
Total or partial loss of coat. No itching and no infection.	Wool slip. Not uncommon and thought due to hormonal factors.	No treatment. Protection from the worst of the weather may be necessary.
BREATHING		
Rapid breathing.	Symptoms may be due to pain, over exercise or overheating. Pneumonia commonly due to bacterial infection eg. Pasteurella. Parasitic Pneumonia due to lungworm infection. Many species could be involved. Jaagsiekte (Pulmonary Adenomatosis) due to virus infection.	Remove source of the stress and the symptoms should resolve quite quickly. Injectable antibiotic. Reduce stress, check ventilation if indoors. Vaccine available for Pasteurella infection. Anthelmintic required. Ivermectin or Levamisole or Fenbendazole among others are effective. No treatment available. Get stock from disease-free sources.
Shallow breathing.	Asleep or in terminal stage of illness.	Check for other symptoms and get vet as necessary.
Coughing.	Respiratory infection eg. Pneumonia due to infection from bacteria, virus or parasite. Inhalation Pneumonia following faulty drenching or dosing.	Antibiotic, anti-inflammatory drugs and mucolytics. Anthelmintic for lungworm. Get vet to check diagnosis. Antibiotic to control secondary infection. Improve drenching technique.

Signs of Disease	Causes	Treatment and Prevention
TEMPERATURE (normal range is 101.5 - 102.5°F)		
Raised.	Usually means infection but may be the result of heat stress or pain.	Check for other symptoms. If in doubt check with the vet. Antiobiotic for infection, pain killers for pain.
Lowered.	Check again. May be incorrect technique or reading. If correct may be terminally ill.	Check for other symptoms eg. diarrhoea. Give symptomatic treatment until a diagnosis is established eg. warm patient up slowly.
DUNG		
Constipation.	Uncommon but may be the sequel to digestion problems or fever.	Consider the primary cause of the problem and give laxative eg. liquid paraffin or epsom salts in bran mash.
Scouring.	Parasitic gastroenteritis ie. worms, many species may be involved. Faecal sample required to make diagnosis.

Chronic Fascioliasis ie. chronic fluke infection. | Dose with anthelmintic and move onto clean pasture.

Dose with anthelmintic preparation specifically for fluke. Drain land and get rid of snail which is the intermediate host. |
Scouring, light in colour.	Ruminal acidosis due to animal having eaten too many concentrates or cereal.	Take off concentrate diet. Give bicarbonate by mouth. Multivitamins and antihistamines may help.
Dung persistently soft.	Johne's Disease due to infection by Mycobacterium johnei.	None. Slaughter all known cases.
Scouring after change of diet or moving onto new pasture.	Nutritional upset due to change of diet or lush pasture.	Increase roughage in diet eg. hay and symptoms will disappear.
Scouring with retarded growth and wool reduced or straight without crimp.	Consider copper or cobalt deficiency. Need blood test for diagnosis.	Give copper or cobalt orally or by injection.
BLOAT		
Bloat ie. abdominal distension of left side of abdomen.	Gas not being belched from rumen. Could be due to obstruction in gullet or failure in the mechanism to allow belching or frothy bloat (more common in adult sheep) where gas and stomach contents are mixed as a froth.

Frothy bloat usually caused by overeating, especially on lucerne or clover. | If bloat due to obstruction remove it or push it down into the stomach. If this is not possible vet will usually insert trocar and cannula to relieve abdominal distention.

If frothy bloat use stomach drench of silicone or vegetable oil preparations. |
| Bloat with distention on both sides of abdomen. | Severe bloat. Animal will be close to death. | May require emergency trocarisation. Get vet ASAP. |

Signs of Disease	Causes	Treatment and Prevention
URINE		
Urinary retention or blockage sometimes with distended abdomen.	Urolithiasis. Not common in adult sheep. Due to calculi blocking the urethra.	Muscle relaxant drugs can help if blockage is only partial. Surgery or euthanasia in severe cases. Salt in diet may be used as prevention. Check diet.
Discoloured urine, often dark red in colour.	Clostridial infection. Animal usually collapsed due to Toxaemia. Copper poisoning due to excessive intake. Rape or other brassica poisoning.	Antibiotic and fluid therapy. Poor prognosis. Vaccinate to prevent. Oral dose of sodium sulphate and ammonium molybdate may help. Remove from source of trouble. Multivitamins may help. Feed hay before putting onto brassica grazing and control amount grazed.
Pain in abdomen; seen as lying down and getting up frequently, teeth grinding and kicking while lying down.	Colic due to bloat, Urolithiasis or intestinal torsion or blockage. Clostridial infections can cause pain eg. Pulpy Kidney.	Muscle relaxants and pain killers may help (plus see above). Clostridial antisera and antibiotic. Vaccinate to prevent.
LAMENESS		
Feet.	Bacterial infection in the foot eg. foot abscess, foot rot or foot scald. Commonly due to fusiformis species or, if abscess, Corynebacteria. Virus infection eg. Foot and Mouth disease (NB. notifiable disease). Bluetongue - inflammation and pain due to swelling above hooves (NB. notifiable disease).	Pare foot where appropriate and dress with topical antibiotic spray. Inject antibiotic where necessary. Keep on dry ground and use foot baths. Check for ulcers in mouth. If in doubt call vet. No effective treatment. Vaccinate.
Limbs.	Injury eg. fracture, nerve damage, puncture wound or strain. Clostridial infection eg. Blackleg. Specific joint infection eg. Erysipelas or C. pyogenes. Tick pyaemia due to Staph. aureus abscesses in the joints and perhaps elsewhere.	All but the most minor may need vet attention. Treat as required by symptoms. Large doses of antibiotic and antisera. Vaccinate to prevent. Antibiotic and good hygiene required. Clean pens and dips. Antibiotic. Tick control can help.
Reluctant to move on all limbs or just forelimbs.	Laminitis ie. inflammation of the lamina of the foot due to bacterial toxins in blood stream or may just be overweight.	Pain killing and anti-inflammatory drugs. Bathe feet in warm water.

Signs of Disease	Causes	Treatment and Prevention
INFERTILITY - FEMALE		
Failure to come into season.	Pregnant.	Vet required to check for any possible pregnancy.
	Low body weight or deficiency disease eg. copper or manganese.	Check diagnosis with blood samples before undertaking any treatment.
	Possible genetic trace infection.	Antibiotic or cull from flock.
	Ovarian problems which, if young sheep, may be congenital.	If treating individual it may be worth trying hormone treatment, but if congenital problem cull from flock.
Abortion.	Infection most likely cause eg. Enzootic Abortion due to Chlamydia. (NB. can cause serious infection in women).	All abortions should be investigated with blood tests and swabs before attempting treatment.
	Toxoplasmosis, Border disease, Campylobacter, Listeriosis, tick borne fever and fungal infections are the most common.	Good hygiene essential at all times. Vaccine available for prevention of Enzootic and Toxoplasmosis. Isolate affected animals until diagnosis is made.
	Isolated cases may be due to poor handling and clumsy management.	Check management.
Vaginal discharge. Clear with or without blood stain.	If pregnant may be about to give birth. Slight discharge may be apparent when in season.	If in doubt get vet to check.
Purulent, smelly discharge with or without afterbirth being retained.	May be primary infection in genital tract or due to retained afterbirth, some of which may be hanging from vulva. Dead lamb(s) may still be retained in uterus.	Antibiotic by injection and/or intro-uterine pessaries or uterine irrigation. Remove retained afterbirth if possible and any retained lambs.
INFERTILITY - MALE		
	Specific infection in the testicle(s).	Better to cull the animal than attempt treatment.
	Deficiency disease eg. vitamin A or zinc.	Vitamin or zinc supplements.
	Orthopaedic problems eg. sore back or legs or pelvis making it difficult for the animal to mount.	Should be self-evident to careful observation. Get vet to check and treat any lameness.
	Sores around sheath or scrotum may inhibit mating. Check for Orf (NB. infectious to people).	Localised treatment with antibiotic may be helpful.

Signs of Disease	Causes	Treatment and Prevention
MASTITIS		
Milk very thick immediately after lambing.	Normal/colostrum.	No action required. Will clear in a day or so.
Clots in milk.	Mild form of Mastitis. Many bacteria might be involved, but probably a Streptococcus.	Intramammary antibiotic required.
Milk very watery and udder often very sore and red.	Acute Mastitis due to E. coli or Pasteurella or Staphylococcus aureus.	Antibiotic both intramammary and injectable.
Udder cold, ewe very ill, blood stained fluid present at teat.	Peracute Mastitis with gangrene. Usually due to Staph. aureus or Pasteurella infection.	May be necessary to amputate teat to allow drainage. Antibiotic, anti-inflammatory drugs and electrolytes may be required. Grave prognosis.
Udder normal temperature but hard, no milk expressed.	Chronic Mastitis. May be just blocked teat canal.	Possibly no effective treatment, but try antibiotic injection. Cull ewe before next lambing season. Get vet to check and unblock if possible.
Red sores over the udder area.	Orf ie. virus infection (NB. infectious to people). Sheep pox (NB. a notifiable disease), (rare) or Dermatophilus infection.	Antibiotic may help. Vaccine available. Antibiotic may be useful in both cases.
BEHAVIOUR		
Loss of appetite.	Any infection causing a rise in temperature. Pain - check for sores in mouth/blisters eg. Foot and Mouth disease (NB. notifiable disease). Check for abdominal pain eg. teeth grinding and grunting.	Check for other symptoms before starting treatment. Treatment depending on cause of pain and definite diagnosis required - see vet.
Slow progressive loss of appetite in pregnant animal and finally recumbency.	Pregnancy Toxaemia due to energy deficiency caused by faulty management.	Glycerol, propylene glycol orally, steroids and anabolic steroid. Abortion may be necessary to save ewe's life. Ensure adequate diet and exercise in last half of pregnancy.
Fairly sudden loss of appetite and then recumbency in later pregnancy and after lambing.	Hypocalcaemia/lack of calcium in circulation.	Give calcium intravenously or under the skin.

Signs of Disease	Causes	Treatment and Prevention
BEHAVIOUR CONTINUED		
Walking in circles and head pressing.	Middle ear infection or Listeriosis.	Antibiotic. Avoid silage feeding. Good hygiene essential.
	Gid (Sturdy) ie. tapeworm cyst in brain.	Surgery to remove cyst. Routine tapeworm dosing of all dogs.
Head pressing with peculiar gait, then recumbency.	Louping Ill due to virus infection.	Antisera may be some use if used early. Vaccine available. Control tick which is inter-mediate host.
Progressive loss of condition with gradual paralysis.	Maedi Visna viral infection.	No cure. Slaughter all affected animals. Blood test is available.
Intense itch with loss of condition despite good appetite, later head raised with lip nibbling.	Scrapie (NB. notifiable disease) due to infection by small virus-like particle.	Slaughter all affected animals.
Fits and foaming at the mouth.	Hypomagnesaemia due to low levels of magnesium in blood stream. Common on lush pasture.	Magnesium injection given under the skin. Feed magnesium rich feed. Restrict time on lush pasture. Magnesium boluses.
SUDDEN DEATH		
Without prior warning.	Anthrax. ie. infection with Bacillus anthracis (NB. notifiable disease and infectious to people).	Rare and usually from contaminated feed.
	Any of the clostridial diseases eg. Braxy or Black disease.	Vaccines are available and very effective.
	Plant poisoning eg. yew or laurel.	Never leave hedge or tree clippings where animals can reach them.
	Hypomagnesaemia (see above).	Prevention can be simple and effective (see above).
	Lightning strike.	Post-mortem should be able to show scorch marks on the skin.

DIAGNOSTIC GUIDE TO LAMB AILMENTS AND TREATMENT

Signs of Disease	Causes	Treatment and Prevention
HEAD AND FACE		
Nasal discharge.	Pneumonia due to virus or bacterial infection.	Antibiotic. Check environment for overcrowding and if indoors, ventilation. If outdoors check shelter provision in inclement weather.
Nasal discharge with blood and pus.	Sheep nasal fly - seen only in the summer.	Ivermectin may be helpful as can be organophosphorus dips.
Ulcers on lips, tongue and dental pad.	Foot and Mouth disease (NB. notifiable disease) but unlikely to be seen only in lambs.	Check for other symptoms eg. blisters on feet. If suspicious inform the vet.
Scabs on lips, also on nostril and eye lids.	Orf ie. infection by Paravaccinia virus (NB. infectious to people).	Topical ointments and sprays can stop secondary bacterial infection. Isolate affected animals. Vaccine available.
Scabs on face ie. around eyes, ears and base of horns.	Facial eczema due to bacterial infection ie. Staphylococcus aureus. Head fly. Photosensitisation may be a factor in summer months.	Antibiotic. Check trough space is adequate. Pour on preparations. Ingestion of St. John's wort or clover may precipitate condition. Move pasture or indoors. Try steroids or antihistamines.
Loss of hair on face especially around eyes.	Ringworm, usually due to Trichophyton verrucosum. Rare. (NB. infectious to people).	Topical antifungal agents.
Salivation and drooling from the mouth.	Virus infection eg. Foot and Mouth disease or Orf (see above). Actinobacillosis ie. bacterial infection in mouth, jaw bone and elsewhere. Colibacillosis ie. watery mouth. Due to infection by E. coli.	See above for Foot and Mouth disease and Orf. Antibiotic or sodium iodide intravenous weekly or potassium iodide orally daily Antibiotic and Metoclopramide and electrolytes. Ensure good colostrum uptake. Good hygiene essential.
EYES		
Watery discharge from one or both eyes.	Entropion ie. inturned eye lid(s).	Easily rectified by vet with minor surgery. If major problem consider breeding programme.
White discharge from one or both eyes sometimes with damage to the surface of the eye.	Infectious Kerato-conjunctivitis due to infection by Rickettsia or Chlamydia organism.	Subconjunctival injection (job for the vet) or topical antibiotic ointment. Control is difficult. Reduce crowding.
Discharge from one eye with or without eye damage.	Consider foreign body in the eye.	Careful search and remove and then administer antibiotic ointment.
Swollen eye lids.	Allergic reaction.	Antihistamines and/or corticosteroids. May have to move pastures.
Eyes dull and lifeless.	Part of any general disease eg. colisepticaemia.	Look for other symptoms and then treat generally.
Yellow colour in white of the eye.	Jaundice usually the result of copper poisoning.	Oral dose of sodium sulphate may help, but generally poor prognosis.

Signs of Disease	Causes	Treatment and Prevention
EYES CONTINUED		
Blindness.	Congenital cataracts. Older lambs - rape poisoning or Cerebrocortical Necrosis. Bracken poisoning.	Nothing practical can be done. Remove from rape field. Inject thiamine in high doses. Remove from source. Antibiotic and thiamine may help.
Membranes of the eye pale or white.	Anaemia due to worms or deficiency of iron or copper in diet. Rape poisoning.	Treat with anthelmintic. Copper given in slow release bolus. Iron by injection or orally. Remove from offending diet.
Membranes of eye dark and congested.	Circulatory difficulties as part of more general disease eg. Pneumonia.	Check for other symptoms and treat for general disease - see vet.
Eyes sunk into eye sockets.	Dehydration usually as the result of scouring.	Electrolytes as fluid replacer and treat the cause of the scour.
EARS		
One or both ears swollen.	Abscess or blood blister.	Drain abscess and give antibiotic. Blood blister leave to reabsorb naturally.
One ear drooping with possible discharge from ear canal.	Bacterial infection, consider Listeriosis.	Antibiotic. If Listeriosis consider source of infection eg. silage. Also practise good hygiene in lambing pen.
SKIN AND FLEECE		
Loss of fleece with scabs and itching.	Sheep scab due to Psoroptic mite infection. Any untreated sheep with infection may be welfare case and owner prosecuted if not attended to.	Dip with approved sheep scab dip. Ensure all safety precautions are observed when dipping.
Loss of fleece with itching. Parasites found.	Lice, ticks and keds could all be involved.	Dip or spray or pour on infected animals with recommended products. May have to be repeated every 10 - 14 days.
Wet staining of wool mostly around rear end with animal distressed.	Blowfly maggots.	Dag the flock ie. clean and clip area of the dock. Dip or spray. Severely affected animals may have to be destroyed.
Excessively long and curly wool with nervous symptoms.	Border disease due to virus infection in the ewe in the first 2-3 months of gestation.	None available. Separate infected and non-infected mothers.
Wrinkled skin with sores.	Zinc deficiency. Rare condition.	Zinc sulphate weekly. Control with zinc fertiliser on pasture.
BREATHING		
Rapid breathing.	Pneumonia commonly due to bacterial infection eg. Pasteurella. Acute infection, young animal often found dead. Stress due to pain, overheating or exercise.	Antibiotic. Reduce stress, check ventilation if indoors. Vaccine available for Pasteurella infection. Remove source of the stress and the symptoms should resolve quickly.
Shallow breathing.	Asleep or in terminal stage of illness.	No action. Check for other symptoms. Get vet.

Signs of Disease	Causes	Treatment and Prevention
BREATHING CONTINUED		
Coughing.	Respiratory disease eg. Pneumonia due to infection.	Antibiotic, anti-inflammatory and mucolytic drugs.
	Unlikely to be lungworm unless in older lambs.	Anthelmintic for lungworm. See vet for diagnosis.
	Inhalation Pneumonia following faulty drenching and dosing.	Antibiotic to control secondary infection. Improve drenching technique.
TEMPERATURE (normal range is 101.5 - 102.5°F)		
Raised.	Usually means infecton but may be the result of stress or pain.	Check for other symptoms. If in doubt check with vet. Antibiotic for infection, pain killers for pain.
Lowered.	Check again, may be incorrect technique or reading.	Raise body temperature with heat lamps or equivalent. Warm air heaters.
	Hypothermia in young lambs is a common killer.	Check for other symptoms eg. diarrhoea.
	May be terminally ill.	
Shivering.	Young lambs with early stages of hypothermia.	See above. If indoors check for draughts. If outdoors are there adequate windbreaks?
DUNG		
Constipation.	Can be one of the symptoms of wet mouth (more commonly diarrhoea). Not uncommon if lamb has not received colostrum.	Check for other symptoms. Liquid paraffin useful 1-2 teaspoonfuls.
Scouring. Young lambs no blood in diarrhoea.	Bacterial infection eg. E. coli which also causes watery mouth symptoms.	Antibiotic and electrolytes. Keep the patient warm. Colostrum essential for prevention as is good hygiene.
Scouring with blood in diarrhoea.	Lamb dysentery due to clostridial infection.	Antibiotic and electrolytes. Keep the patient warm.
Older lambs with diarrhoea, perhaps some blood.	Coccidiosis usually infection with Eimeria species.	Oral antibacterials eg. amprolium or sulphadimidine. Avoid overcrowding and wet areas. Prophylactic in feed medication can be used.
Older lambs with diarrhoea, no blood.	Parasitic gastroenteritis ie. worms. These include Haemonchus, Ostertagia, Trichstongylus, Oesophagostomum and Nematodiaris species.	Anthelmintic to all affected animals. Drench ewes prior to lambing and move to clean pasture ie. pasture not used by sheep the previous year.

Signs of Disease	Causes	Treatment and Prevention
BLOAT		
Bloat ie. abdominal distention of left side of abdomen.	Gas not being belched from rumen. Could be obstruction in gullet or failure in the mechanism to allow belching or frothy bloat .Uncommon in young lambs, except those bottle fed. Older lambs due to overeating, especially lucerne or clover.	Stomach drench silicone or oil preparation. Get vet to check diet. As above and restict grazing of suspect pasture.
Bloat with distention on both sides of abdomen.	Severe bloat. Animal will be close to death.	May require emergency trocarisation. Get vet ASAP.
Swelling under belly at the navel.	Navel infection. Umbilical hernia.	Antibiotic. Dip navel at birth with iodine or spray with antibiotic. If small no action required. If large surgery may be needed.
URINE		
Urinary retention or blockage sometimes with distended abdomen.	Urolithiasis. Common in housed lambs on concentrate feed. Due to calculi (stone) blocking urethra.	Muscle relaxant drugs may help. Surgery or euthanasia for severe cases. Check diet. Salt in diet may help prevent new cases.
Discoloured urine often dark red in colour.	Clostridial infection. Animal usually collapsed due to Toxaemia.	Antibiotic and fluid therapy. Poor prognosis. Vaccinate as prevention.
Pain in abdomen; seen as lying down and getting up frequently, teeth grinding and kicking while lying down.	Colic due to bloat or Urolithiasis. Clostridial infections can cause pain eg. Pulpy Kidney or Lamb Dysentery.	Muscle relaxants and/or pain killers (plus see above). Clostridial antisera and antibiotic. Vaccinate as prevention.
LAMENESS		
Feet.	Bacterial infection in the foot eg. foot abscess, foot rot or foot scald. Commonly due to fusiformis species, or if abscess Corynebacteria. Virus infection eg. Foot and Mouth disease (NB. notifiable disease).	Pare foot where appropriate and dress with topical spray. Inject antibiotic. Keep on dry ground and use foot baths. Check for ulcers in mouth. Call vet.
Deformed limbs.	Rickets due to a dietary imbalance of calcium/phosphorus and vitamin D.	Oral or injectable calcium/phosphorus and vitamin D preparations. Check and maintain adequate diet.
Stiff limbs.	Vitamin E/selenium deficiency.	Vitamin E and selenium injections. Nutritional supplements.

Signs of Disease	Causes	Treatment and Prevention
LAMENESS CONTINUED		
Limbs - general.	Injury eg. fracture, nerve damage, puncture wounds or strain.	All but most minor may need vet attention. Treat as required by symptoms.
	Clostridial infection eg. Blackleg.	Large doses of antibiotic and antiserum. Vaccinate to prevent.
	Specific joint infection eg. Erysipelas or C. pyogenes.	Antibiotic and good hygiene required. Clean pens and dips. Dip navels at birth.
	Tick pyaemia due to Staph. aureus abscesses in the joints and maybe elsewhere.	Antibiotic. Tick control can help.
BEHAVIOUR		
Loss of appetite.	Any infection causing a rise in temperature.	Check for other symptoms before starting treatment.
	Pain - check mouth for sores, check for abdominal pain.	Treatment depends on cause of pain. Pain killers, anti-inflammatory drugs and antibiotic may all be helpful.
	Pain causing lameness unlikely to cause loss of appetite.	
Dull and weak with low rectal temperature.	Hypothermia due to inadequate shelter or lack of food or both.	Warm gently. Feed with stomach tube if not sucking/Intra Peritomeal glucose injection. Ensure adequate shelter for ewes and lambs. Make sure lamb gets enough colostrum.
Nervous signs eg. twisted head and neck 'star gazing.'	Daft Lamb Disease ie. congenital disease of Border Leicester Sheep.	No treatment. Review breeding programme.
Lambs born weak with tremors and wool abnormalities.	Border disease due to viral infection.	No treatment. Isolate all infected ewes from unaffected.
Blindness and walking in circles.	Cerebrocortical Necrosis due to thiamine deficiency.	High levels of thiamine by injection.
Walking in circles and head pressing.	Middle ear infection or Listeriosis.	Antibiotic. Avoid silage feeding. Good hygiene important.
	Gid (Sturdy) ie. tapeworm cyst in brain.	Surgery to remove cyst. Routine tapeworm dosing of all dogs.
Head pressing with peculiar gait, then recumbency.	Louping Ill due to virus infection.	Antisera may be some use if used early. Vaccine available. Control tick which is the intermediate host.
Uncoordinated limb movements and swaying.	Swayback. Due to a congenital copper deficiency.	Nothing much helps to treat clinical cases. Control by giving pregnant ewes copper injections or slow release copper bolus.

Signs of Disease	Causes	Treatment and Prevention
SUDDEN DEATH		
Without prior warning.	Anthrax ie. infection with Bacillus anthracis (NB. notifiable disease and infectious to people).	Rare. The source of infection is usually contaminated feed.
	Any of the clostridial diseases eg. Lamb Dysentery or Pulpy Kidney.	Vaccines are available and very effective.
	Plant poisoining eg. yew or laurel.	Never leave hedge or tree clippings where animals can reach them.
	Lightning strike.	Post-mortem should be able to show scorch marks on skin.

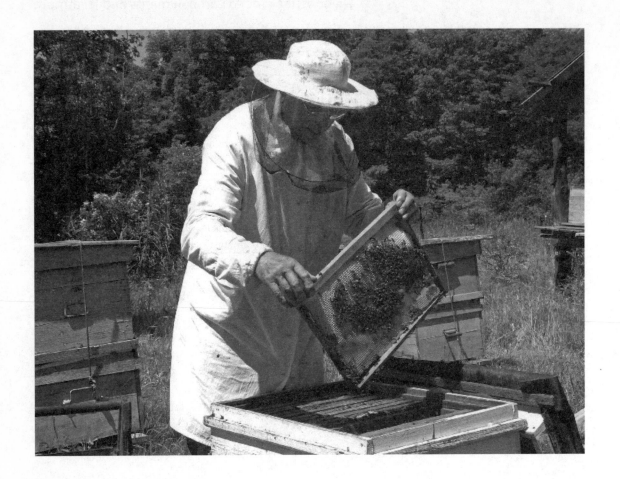

Chapter Seven

THE TROUBLE WITH BEES

By Paul Peacock

As I write this there is a most interesting parallel. In 1894 some mites entered the US from Mexico attached to bee colonies, hidden deep in the trachea of the animals. Within twenty years the entire population of British bees were all but wiped out. Acarapis woodi is a parasite which lives in the breathing holes (trachaea) of adult bees, causing them to suffocate. In the UK almost the whole population of black bees was lost, though pockets did remain from which pioneers are now trying to find out exactly what happened.

It was not until the 1920s that we learnt that the culprit was a parasite. Until then the disease had been a mystery. It seems to be the lot of beekeepers to suffer mysterious and strange threats to their stock. Being a beekeeper in 1904 when the disease first appeared on the Isle of White (it was known as Isle of White Disease), must have been remarkably like today; both bewildering and worrying.

All the bees we know in the UK today have been bred specially, mostly by a group of monks under the guidance of the famous Brother Adam. The entire population of bees was replaced in a fairly short period, which just goes to show that there are solutions out there if we care to look.

It has to be said, however, that the bee has lived unhindered on the earth for many hundreds of millions of years. For the species to suffer at least two catastrophes in only the last hundred must show the impact that man has had on them.

Compare a bee to a varroa mite. The bee reproduces and therefore changes or modifies its genetic material once every three or so years. A varroa mite does so every few weeks. Useful mutations for the varroa mite (such as resistance to treatments) can be much more quickly introduced into the general population than in a bee where mutations to the genetic material can only be passed on every few years. Consequently bees do far more readily fall prey to devastating diseases.

Moreover, the bee gene pool is a shallow one. Each hive is genetically more or less an individual. So, with the sharing of genes from within a colony, not much active evolution goes on. But bees do evolve, which they did when the wild population was wiped out in the early years of last century.

The Importance Of Regular Checking

Unfortunately these days it is not possible to have a colony of bees simply left to their own devices. They will die, and the beekeeper is now faced with the need for constant vigilance to maintain colony strength and health. Beekeepers need to be fully versed in the techniques of assessing varroa mite numbers and must understand the impact of this mite on the colony.

Keeping bees healthy is a matter of regular checking in the first instance. You are looking for a healthy queen and full brood combs with few (if any) holes in them. You are looking for strong flying bees who look healthy, with as many returning to the hive as there are leaving it.

Then you are counting varroa mites and looking for certain tell tale signs – bees holding their wings in a 'K' shape, bees being listless and horrid deformities caused by varroa.

Another important skill is to understand when and how best to feed your bees. If they are unable to forage, or you have taken honey, it is important to get food into the colony, though every beekeeper will tell you there is no substitute for a good nectar flow. You can't keep bees on sugar syrup alone and it is simply greedy to do so!

An Important Rule

• Bees can withstand one problem fairly easily.
• They can just about cope with two for a short period.
• They will die if they have three problems to deal with.

Heavy varroa infestation, a lack of food and cold weather will kill bees. Similarly, varroa, nosema and rainy weather will kill bees. Heavy pesticide presence, and any other problems combined will kill also your bees.

Varroa

You will notice that all the problems facing bees involve varroa at some point. Beekeepers first thought the problem of the tiny mites that invade brood cells at the larvae stage, deforming the developing bees, could be controlled by insecticides. However it wasn't long before the treatments produced strains of varroa mites completely immune to the chemicals used to treat them. Consequently beekeepers have developed a number of different methods other than blanket treatments with chemicals. These control methods are not designed to remove all the mites from the colony, but to keep them at a level at which the bees can cope.

These methods have completely changed the pattern and, in a real sense the methods, of beekeeping. If you used to keep bees ten years ago and were suddenly returning to the craft then you would find the practice quite different. The hive itself is different these days. First of all it has a wire mesh floor. When the mites fall off the bee or comb they now fall right out of the hive and never get back in.

There tends not to be a bee escape mechanism at the top of the hive and frequently no crown board either.

A regular way of reducing mite numbers is to take advantage of the fact that mites prefer to enter drone brood. A blank frame on which workers will make drone comb is placed on the hive and then, when you have the grubs capped, the comb is discarded and a good number of mites with it.

There are a number of ways of counting varroa mites. You can take an area of brood when the larvae are at the pink eye stage and count the number of mites on them. This gives an idea but it is not easy, is certainly invasive and has limited use.

The most reliable way of estimating the total number of mites is to count how many fall out of the hive through the wire mesh floor. For every mite that falls through there are prob-

ably 30 to 100 in the hive, depending on the time of the year.

What you need to do is calculate an average 'daily fall.' So, if over 14 days you collected 96 mites this means you have 96 divided by 14 or 6.8 mites falling per day.

There is a fairly complex mathematical calculation to work out how many mites are in the hive, but the following rule of thumb is a good guide.

Between May and August multiply the daily average fall by 30. In August, September and October multiply it by 100.

If the varroa population you have calculated gets to 500 mites it won't be long before they multiply to 1000 – which is said to be the critical level.

If your total estimate is higher than 500 mites I would think about treating and if it is over 800 then treat right away. However, you need to be aware of treatment resistance, but more of that later.

You must conduct regular inspections and counting of varroa mite numbers will allow you to make sensible judgements about your hives. The use of drone brood sacrifice and treatments with chemicals will ensure varroa numbers are at their lowest.

Apistan

The government has now outlawed the sale of Apistan. This was a treatment that came in strips hung between the frames and was used in late September each year regardless of the number of mites in the hive, or whenever you found a lot of mites in the hive. Tests in the USA and Canada have shown that Apistan is better than any other chemical at killing varroa, but mites do acquire resistance over time and it is because of this resistance that the product has been withdrawn. Now Thymol, which so far has had no possibility of any resistance implications, is used. Thymol is an essential oil that comes in crystals that dissolve in methylated spirits.

There are many ways to administer Thymol, but it is mostly done in strips hung between the frames like Apistan. You can also buy a frame with a built in reservoir for the crystals themselves and you can add it in a low concentration to winter sugar feed too. Thymol also works to reduce fungal problems and helps with Acarine and Chalkbrood. Apiguard is a readily available product containing thymol.

Oxalic acid is administered only once a year in December when it is cold – so you have to be quick. The substance kills up to 90% of the mites and is dissolved in sugar syrup at the rate of 3.5%. In the brood box you have to trickle the syrup onto the frames at the rate of 5ml (ish) per frame. It is convenient to buy a syringe to do this.

You cover all the bees and they will release their dead mites over the next month or so. It is important that you apply oxalic acid when all the brood larvae are gone, which is why this procedure takes place in December. The queen will stop laying when the first frost arrives, and so three weeks later there will be no brood.

Formic acid at 65% is used during the summer months and in spring using a specially bought evaporator. It will evaporate directly into the cells of brood and kill mites. You need to remove honey first because it will be tainted and the bees will need to be fed syrup too. The varroa floor should be closed and you should only use this treatment when the temperature

is between 5°C and 20°C. Higher temperatures will cause too much evaporation and thus kill bees.

There are other treatments such as dusting the bees with sugar, triggering a cleaning response which does knock off some of the mites too, but the major common remedies are the ones beekeepers should be concentrating on.

Keep yourself abreast of new developments in bee health as new remedies are appearing all the time. There are movements to create a special entrance that knocks off the mites as the bees push themselves through as well as improved treatments and the development of bee strains that clean the mite away most effectively.

Colony Collapse Syndrome

Massive colony losses around the world from during 2004 and without real explanation have rocked beekeepers. This particular problem has spread around the world very quickly and it is believed that 30% of colonies have been killed each year for the last three years. The problem has been referred to as colony collapse syndrome and is probably a combination of a number of factors; varroa, pesticides, acute bee paralysis virus and a new and worrying form of the bee dysentery called Nosema.

Nosema Apis

Normally nosema (caused by a species called Nosema apis) is quite visible because the bees empty their guts all over the hive and the place is a complete mess – imagine 10,000 bees with diarrhoea! Consequently it is possible to treat for Nosema apis because you can see when it is happening.

The recognised treatment is Fumidil B (now

often called Fumigilin). Complete disinfecting of the hive is recommended together with moving the bees to a new hive where there are no spores to be ingested.

A preventative treatment, Protofil, is being tested and is said to have an efficiency of between 70% and 90% at keeping colonies clear.

One important factor is to try to get new colonies that are certified free of the disease, because otherwise you will be unlikely to see them develop into a strong mature colony.

Nosema ceranae

The new form of nosema is completely invisible because the bees don't get diarrhoea; they simply become sicker and sicker and when the female workers leave the hive they are usually too ill to get back. They die in rain showers, on leaves and in flowers and the colony reduces in number at an alarming rate.

Inside the hive the situation is much the same. You can see the affected workers walking around the hive with their wings at jaunty angles and, unable to fly, they stop feeding. A colony can die within a week. This and high varroa load can also be a trigger to the rapid death of the colony.

The agent of this disease, Nosema ceranae, is a unicellular parasite akin to other dysentery causing creatures in most other animals, including humans. However, you are not at risk yourself from this particular parasite. You will find it described as a fungus in much of the literature.

Nosema ceranae can also be treated with Fumidil B. The bad news in the case of both Nosema apis and Nosema cerenae is that Fumigil B is banned in Europe and when supplies run out it might be that we are also not allowed to use it in the UK. Thymol has been

described as an effective method of fighting the disease, but this is based only on hearsay evidence. The big question, however, is when do you know you have it as a problem? The answer is, you don't.

For the moment a springtime, summertime and autumn feed of sugar syrup with Fumidil B will help keep the hive clear. To a certain extent it also stops the transmission of the problem to other colonies.

Constant vigilance and research are our best hope in this fight, but it will be some time before we get a real and permanent answer to this problem.

Foulbrood

There are two kinds of foulbrood; American (AFB) and European (EFB). Both of them are caused by a bacterium that affects developing larvae. AFB kills pupating larvae in capped cells, although they will have become infected when very young; EFB usually becomes evident before the cells are capped. In AFB the brood comb is blackened and the cappings are sunken a little because of the death and decay of the contents. With EFB the cells are uncapped and there is an acrid smell as well as decaying watery and ropey cell contents.

AFB is a notifiable disease and your local Bee Inspector will come and confirm the diagnosis. If he is sure about the presence of the disease the colony and hive will have to be burned and everything else disinfected.

The basic test for foulbrood is to touch the cell with a match and pull it out. The larva has been turned to a runny soup by the bacterium and you can pull out a gooey string of cell contents.

EFB can be treated with antibiotics. It can also

appear and then disappear just as quickly, but the spores are there in the hive. You can buy a testing kit to confirm their presence, but in many cases the colony will not get rid of the problem and will have to be destroyed. A similar kit exists for AFB, but the sole remedy here will be the destruction of the colony.

Chalkbrood And Stonebrood

These are fungal diseases of the hive. Chalkbrood can be controlled by increasing ventilation and requeening to increase the strength of the colony. Removal of the frames will benefit too. It occurs in the spring and is less prevalent since the introduction of varroa floors. Once the larva has been killed its body is consumed by the fungus and it turns white, looking rather like chalk.

The brood 'rattles' in the cells and in advanced cases the workers cut the cappings and throw the mummies out of the hive. White carcases at the entrance to the hive are a good indication of chalk brood.

Stonebrood is the bee equivalent of aspergillosis, which causes a respiratory complaint in humans, birds and animals. The larva turns black and is solidified so that it is difficult to crush, hence the name. These two diseases are not that common in the UK. They can be treated or kept at bay with Thymol preparations with some success, but this is far from an effective treatment.

Acarine

We have already mentioned this in the introduction to this chapter. It is a mite (Acarapis woodi) that infects the air passages (trachea) of adult bees, which become increasingly less able to cope with the lack of oxygen.

The female mite lays eggs in the tubules and the larvae escape and wait around on the frames looking to find a newly emerged bee. They then enter the new worker who will stay in the hive for another 22 days. As soon as they enter they start laying eggs and the cycle of infection increases.

The mite causes the bees to crawl about and you find wings dislocated into in a 'K' position. There will be few fliers and the colony will be in danger of collapse. It is treated with menthol crystals, which you can buy in evaporators. The treatment is temperature sensitive; too hot and you will get too much evaporation, and the bees will vacate the hive. Keep the treatment up for a month at 20°C and you will, on the whole, have dealt with the problem. Some people have used oil of wintergreen to the same effect. Make sure the hive is closed up – no varroa floor etc. Do not use these substances when the bees are collecting honey as there will be a real taint.

'Grease patties' have been used to control this mite. Two parts caster sugar to one part by weight of lard made into little cakes confuse the mite larvae and they cannot find new young bees because they all 'smell' alike. Sometimes people mix some menthol crystals into the patties. The bees eat the patty and it is an effective control.

Sacbrood

This is a viral disease of brood in the late spring when the number of pupating bee larvae is greater than the number of adult bees. The larva dies in the capped cell and turns to liquid, except for the exo-skeleton, which resembles a slipper when pulled out. About a third of colonies exhibit some form of sacbrood infestation. Workers eventually pull them out of the hive and become ill themselves, but they do not pass on the virus to other young because they stop feeding them. The disease can be recognised in much the same way as AFB, but when you pull the contents you get the slipper carcase.

Mice And Birds And Men

In the winter mice raid colonies and eat comb. For some reason they do not disturb wintering bees and so can cause quite a problem, eating honey, destroying comb and so on. They can be prevented by using a mouse guard at the entrance to the hive. This is a piece of aluminium with holes in it that only bees can pass through.

Birds, particularly woodpeckers, can cause havoc with the hive, burrowing through boxes and chilling the bees. This is best stopped by a tarpaulin over the hive and constant vigilance.

Precaution is also needed against vandalism, which can have very devastating results.

Wax Moth

The wax moth causes no end of havoc with stored honeycomb. The grubs tunnel into the wax and honey dribbles everywhere and is lost. The whole frame will be devoured. You can treat by making sure the moth cannot get to stored combs. The moth doesn't like acetic acid, and you can fumigate the frames with sulphur dioxide. This has to be done in a closed system and the treatment is good for other diseases too. Paradochlorobenzine (PCB) is no longer allowed for use against wax moth.
You can also get wax moth traps that have some effect, but are not 100% guaranteed.

Chilled Brood

This is a problem caused by brood that has

been allowed to cool for too long. You should not work in the hive until the temperature approaches 20°C at least. Keeping the frames in the cold air will kill them. Damage to hives will also kill bees in the winter if it becomes too cold for too long. However, bees do well with a varroa floor – it is primarily draughts and rain that chills them.

Induced Dysentery

If you feed brown sugar or weak syrup, which can then ferment, or the honey is not fully mature, you can induce dysentery. This is not a disease but the fault of the beekeeper. The problem is related to starvation. Bees can die of starvation when there is a lot of food around them. They must have at least a full super of capped honey left with them for the winter, but preferably one and a half – around 20kg of honey. Honey is the best food for bees and they should be given sugar syrup on top of this in the autumn to give then plenty of chance to store it properly.

Wasps

If your colony is under stress or has reduced numbers there will be fewer guard bees. These bees will attack any intruder, but if the entrance is too wide they have a big problem. You can narrow the entrance to give the guard bees a fighting chance. Wasps are particularly problematic, and they will not only kill bees, brood and take honey, but they might also bring infections into the hive. You can deal with wasps by closing down the entrance to a minimum (1cm) and using wasp traps which will soon become full.

Small Hive Beetle

This has come from South Africa and is a notifiable disease. A beetle, Aethina tumida, will eat its way through the hive and an infestation will cause the bee colony to vacate. There is debate as to how much damage the beetle actually does in the different parts of the world. Much of this depends on the house clearing traits of the bees. Maintaining good colony strength seems to be the best way to keep this under control, but even good colonies have fallen to small hive beetle. For the sake of other colonies they and the hive should be destroyed completely.

Poisoning

Bees that have been sprayed with insecticide or have collected pollen and nectar from sprayed crops often show bizarre behaviour. They might spin round and round until they die. They often have a distended proboscis. You cannot do anything for them but you can report the problem along with samples of pollen which will help to pinpoint the origin of the problem – though there isn't much you can do then either.

If you have lost a significant number of flying bees you can feed the colony and close down the entrance to mitigate robbing and hope there is enough time left for the newly emerging bees to get themselves to a reasonable nectar flow.

Other Viral Diseases

There are a number of diseases related to viruses which come to the fore when there are other infections happening. There is little to be done about them at the moment. Perhaps the most important is the acute bee paralysis virus, where the bees simply do not move. This is the only virus that is found active in healthy colonies and as such has been implicated in colony collapse disorder.

Index

Cattle

Chicken

Turkey

Goat

Pig

Sheep

Bees

A GUIDE TO TRADITIONAL PIG KEEPING
BY CAROL HARRIS

Whether you want to keep pigs for profit or pleasure, this comprehensive book includes all aspects of traditional pig keeping including choosing the right breed, housing, feeding, stockmanship, ailments, breeding, showing, pigs as pets, sales and marketing and includes a section dedicated to butchering and processing, including making sausages and other recipes. There is a huge resource section too, making this the number one title for the traditional pig keeper.

ISBN 9781904871606

THE SHEEP BOOK FOR SMALLHOLDERS
BY TIM TYNE

This key text covers all the essential information needed to care for your flock on a small scale. Split up into the shepherd's calendar each section covers, in great detail, breeds, housing, feeding, pasture management, stock management, breeding, lambing and obstetrics, ailments, slaughter, butchering, sales, showing, shearing and training your sheep dog, plus a unique section devoted to processing the fleece, including wool spinning and weaving. Combined with an invaluable resource section and appendices, this book is the ultimate shepherd's companion and ideal for both the novice and more experienced sheep keeper, dealing with real things in a way that will inspire ordinary people to believe that they really can do it.

ISBN 9781904871644

NOT JUST FOR CHRISTMAS
BY JANICE HOUGHTON-WALLACE

Heritage turkeys are ideal for small scale farming as they show a higher level of immunity to disease and stress over their commercial counterparts. This beautifully presented and highly acclaimed book puts the turkey back where it belongs and covers its illustrious history, the breeds, housing, equipment, breeding, feeding, development, ailments, legislation, sales and marketing, processing, despatching for the table, exhibition birds and turkeys as pets.

ISBN 9781904871187

RAISING CHICKENS FOR EGGS AND MEAT
BY MIKE WOOLNOUGH

A realistic and honest no-nonsense guide covering all aspects of looking after your chooks, from the joys of seeing your first chicks hatch, caring for them and helping them develop into happy and healthy birds, to finally seeing them safely and humanely dispatched. It intentionally avoids the rose tinted image of keeping chickens and tells it 'how it is.' The book also covers breeds, housing, ailments, nutrition, culling and butchering, making it a realistic introduction to this fast growing pastime and ensuring that any prospective chicken keeper is fully aware of their responsibilities to their birds.

ISBN 9781904871279

AN INTRODUCTION TO KEEPING CATTLE
BY PETER KING

This book is aimed at anyone considering keeping cattle on a small scale for either hobby or profit. With the emphasis very much on the conservation of rare and native breeds the contents include selection, day to day management, nutrition and grazing, housing, breeding, showing, keeping a family cow, cattle ailments, dairying and sales and marketing, making this the essential reference book for anyone considering keeping cattle.

ISBN 9781904871392

RAISING GOATS - MEAT, DAIRY, FIBRE
BY FELICITY STOCKWELL

Goats are one of the most practical additions to any smallholding or large garden. As well as endearing and sociable they are also highly practical and there is a breed to suit every location and environment. This book is aimed at anyone from the first time goat keeper to those thinking of developing a small commercial enterprise in the 21st century. It covers choosing the right breed, general care, maintenance, housing, feeding and dietary requirements, land management, showing, keeping goats as pets and dealing with routine and emergency veterinary care. Dairying, cheese, milking, shearing and spinning fibre, production of meat and skins for home use and direct selling are all covered as well as legal requirements and compliance with Defra and animal health issues, plus a detailed resource section.

ISBN 9781904871675

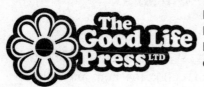

The Good Life Press Ltd.
PO Box 536
Preston
PR2 9ZY
01772 652693

The Good Life Press publishes a wide range of titles for the smallholder, farmer and country dweller as well as HOME FARMER, the monthly magazine for anyone who wants to grab a slice of the good life - whether they live in the country or the city.

Other titles of interest:

A Guide to Traditional Pig Keeping by Carol Harris
An Introduction to Keeping Sheep by J. Upton/D. Soden
Build It! by Joe Jacobs
Build It!..with Pallets by Joe Jacobs
Craft Cider Making by Andrew Lea
First Buy a Field by Rosamund Young
Flowerpot Farming by Jayne Neville
Grow and Cook by Brian Tucker
How to Butcher Livestock and Game by Paul Peacock
Making Country Wines, Ales and Cordials by Brian Tucker
Making Jams and Preserves by Diana Sutton
Precycle! by Paul Peacock
Showing Sheep by Sue Kendrick
Talking Sheepdogs by Derek Scrimgeour
The Bread and Butter Book by Diana Sutton
The Cheese Making Book By Paul Peacock
The Pocket Guide to Wild Food by Paul Peacock
The Polytunnel Companion by Jayne Neville
The Sausage Book by Paul Peacock
The Frugal Life by Piper Terrett
The Sheep Book for Smallholders by Tim Tyne
The Smoking and Curing Book by Paul Peacock
The Medicine Garden by Rachel Corby
The Urban Farmer's Handbook by Paul Peacock
Raising Chickens for Eggs and Meat by Mike Woolnough
Jack Hargreaves - A Portrait by Paul Peacock
The Secret Life of Cows by Rosamund Young

www.goodlifepress.co.uk
www.homefarmer.co.uk